97
Favorite Foods
Every Senior
Should Eat

Publisher's Note

This book is intended for general information only. It does not constitute medical, legal, or financial advice or practice. The editors of FC&A have taken careful measures to ensure the accuracy and usefulness of the information in this book. While every attempt has been made to assure accuracy, errors may occur. Some websites, addresses, and telephone numbers may have changed since printing. We cannot guarantee the safety or effectiveness of any advice or treatments mentioned. Readers are urged to consult with their professional financial advisors, lawyers, and health care professionals before making any changes.

Any health information in this book is for information only and is not intended to be a medical guide for self-treatment. It does not constitute medical advice and should not be construed as such or used in place of your doctor's medical advice. Readers are urged to consult with their health care professionals before undertaking therapies suggested by the information in this book, keeping in mind that errors in the text may occur as in all publications and that new findings may supersede older information.

The publisher and editors disclaim all liability (including any injuries, damages, or losses) resulting from the use of the information in this book.

Then God said, "I give you every seed-bearing plant on the face of the whole earth and every tree that has fruit with seed in it. They will be yours for food."
— *Genesis 1:29 (NIV)*

Table of contents

Nutritional know-how: Discover the hidden power of food

Eat to beat disease: Kitchen cures that help your body heal

Headaches & Migraines. **172**

Heart disease **180**

Heartburn **194**

High blood pressure **201**

Sarcopenia **304**

Sinusitis **314**

Skin cancer **319**

Stress & Anxiety **323**

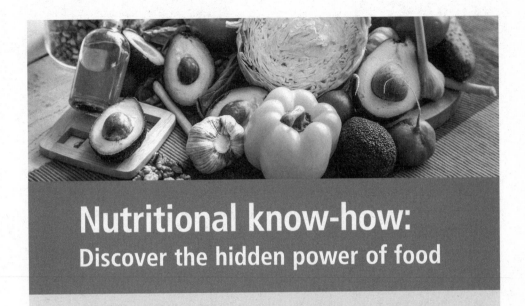

Nutritional know-how:
Discover the hidden power of food

You would never pour any random liquid into your car's gas tank. So why would you fill your body with a haphazard assortment of fuel?

Take some time to learn about the basic components of food — protein, carbohydrates, fiber, fats, vitamins, and minerals. Then discover the healing power of phytochemicals, probiotics, and water. Learn to read food labels and start to understand nutritional building blocks, and you can assemble a menu that will satisfy not only your body but your soul as well.

Help for healthy eating

6 easy switcheroos turn the tables on poor nutrition

Every day you're faced with food choices. And since you eat well over 1,000 meals a year — that's a lot of choices. What drives your decisions could mean the difference between a long, healthy life and one filled with chronic conditions and life-threatening diseases. Learn more about why you eat what you eat and how you can make simple — but effective — changes.

Taste tops the list. Not surprisingly, taste is the No. 1 reason you choose the foods you eat. After all, who can resist sugary sweets, salty snacks, and high-fat fare? Try this easy fix the next time you crave something salty — reach for 10 baked tortilla chips and a half cup of salsa, a low-fat, low-cal alternative.

And to help the young people in your life develop good eating habits, give them healthy treats instead of sugary snacks.

One study shows that if children are frequently offered healthy foods — even those they don't like — they're more likely to get used to them and eat them throughout their life.

Price must be nice. Some people think they can't afford to eat healthy. A recent survey by the International Food Information Council found that cost is the second most-important factor people look at in deciding what to eat. But consider this — an adult can satisfy fruit and vegetable recommendations from the *Dietary Guidelines for Americans* for an average cost of $2 to $2.50 daily. That's less than a bag of potato chips.

Convenience is key. A drive-thru or ready-to-eat meal beats cooking over a hot stove any day, especially if you're juggling work, children, and activities. But those foods aren't always the most nutritious. Satisfy your craving for convenience by freezing leftovers for a later meal or ordering a healthy takeout dish of sauteed chicken and vegetables.

Habits are hard to break. If you feast on bacon or pork sausage for breakfast every morning or can't pass up dessert after dinner every night, you've developed a food habit — and regrettably, not a good one. Studies show that new habits can take 10 weeks or longer to form. Start small, like eating turkey bacon for breakfast or a piece of fruit for dessert. Give yourself the freedom to splurge every now and then.

Regional fare rules. In the South, it's biscuits and gravy. Up North, it's buffalo wings. No matter where you grew up or where you live now, regional cuisine is hard to pass up. Keep the high-fat and fried foods to a minimum. And try to make healthy substitutions, like fresh peaches instead of peach cobbler.

Comfort foods dominate plates. For some, it's a big bowl of ice cream. For others, a platter of fried chicken. No matter how sad or stressed out you feel, emotional eating can lead to overeating and obesity.

> More than a third of Americans over age 20 are obese. Twenty million women and 10 million men suffer from a dangerous eating disorder at some time in their life. And nearly every person in America gets more salt than they should, contributing to up to 40% of all cases of high blood pressure.

Learn to manage your emotions by taking a walk, talking to a friend, or doing something productive. Quench your craving for comfort foods occasionally, not daily.

A host of other reasons, from medical conditions to social engagements, can drive your food decisions. Whatever the reason, make it your goal to blend nutrient-rich meals into your daily diet, and you'll be on your way to a healthier life.

Chew on this: Top sources of calories in the average diet

Americans eat and drink about 2,569 calories a day. As you can see, most of these come from unhealthy sources. Focus on switching out your empty calories for nutritious alternatives.

Vegetables & fruits
8%

Dairy
8%

Flour & cereal products
24%

Sweeteners
16%

Fats & oils, including dairy fat
23%

Meat, eggs, & nuts
21%

New food label cuts the confusion

You no longer have to be a nutrition expert to read the hidden messages on a food label. Thanks to the Food and Drug Administration (FDA), the newly revised Nutrition Facts label on all foods will be easier to read and understand. Plus, shoppers can rest assured that the updated information is based on the latest dietary research.

A food label is like an atlas — it contains information that can guide you from an unhealthy lifestyle to one filled with sound nutrition. Just like a map, you can use food labels to prepare your trips to the supermarket and plan your meals to ensure you arrive at your destination — optimal health. Here's how the new label will help.

Ends confusion over serving size. New requirements will reflect the amount of food people actually eat today as opposed to 25 years ago when labels were first introduced. For instance, manufacturers typically labeled a 20-ounce soda as 2.5 servings with 110 calories per serving. Most people would miss the servings per container and think the entire soda contained 110 calories.

That's one of the hidden messages you'll no longer have to figure out. From now on, a 20-ounce soda will list its entire calorie content — 275 calories for some — and be labeled as one serving, since people typically drink a bottle that size in one sitting. The number of calories will be listed in bold using a larger print size.

Makes nutrition data easier to read. The percentage of daily values (DV) help shoppers calculate nutrient information more easily. The label will continue to include the daily value percentages for iron and calcium. It will add nutritional data for vitamin D and potassium because many Americans don't get enough of these critical nutrients.

As a general guide, 5% DV or less of a nutrient per serving is considered low, and 20% DV or more of a nutrient per serving is considered high.

Highlights added sugar. You won't be fooled by long, complicated sugar names any longer. In the past, manufacturers listed the scientific names of added sugars, and you had no way of knowing how much the product contained. The new food labels will list the total amount of added sugars in grams. While added sugar and naturally occurring sugar are similar chemically, foods loaded with added sugar deliver little to no nutrients. So if your favorite cereal has 10 grams of added sugar, you'll know it's not the healthiest choice.

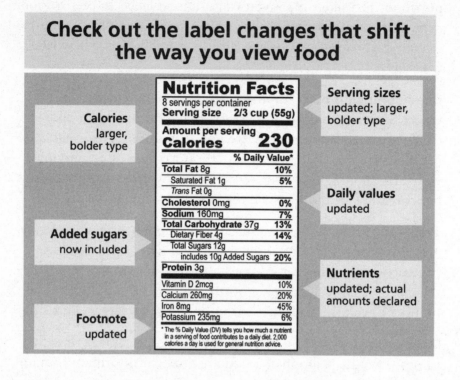

Check out the label changes that shift the way you view food

Calories
larger, bolder type

Added sugars
now included

Footnote
updated

Nutrition Facts
8 servings per container
Serving size   2/3 cup (55g)

Amount per serving
Calories   230

% Daily Value*

Total Fat 8g	**10%**
Saturated Fat 1g	**5%**
Trans Fat 0g	
Cholesterol 0mg	**0%**
Sodium 160mg	**7%**
Total Carbohydrate 37g	**13%**
Dietary Fiber 4g	**14%**
Total Sugars 12g	
includes 10g Added Sugars	**20%**
Protein 3g	
Vitamin D 2mcg	10%
Calcium 260mg	20%
Iron 8mg	45%
Potassium 235mg	6%

* The % Daily Value (DV) tells you how much a nutrient in a serving of food contributes to a daily diet. 2,000 calories a day is used for general nutrition advice.

Serving sizes
updated; larger, bolder type

Daily values
updated

Nutrients
updated; actual amounts declared

7 scary food additives you're eating now

Food companies used an FDA loophole to introduce new food additives that may not be safe, claim public health groups. Food companies deny this, and say ensuring safe products is in their own best interest. So what counts as a food additive, and what does all this mean for you?

Know your additives. During the making or processing of a food, extra ingredients may be added. Any that become part of the final product or affect its characteristics are called food additives. Additives can be natural — like vinegar, salt, or spices — or manmade chemicals — like artificial colors and preservatives.

Additives are used for many good reasons.

- add nutrients
- keep the product fresh

- prevent foodborne illness
- help process or prepare the product
- preserve texture
- enhance color or flavor

Compounds from packaging or other sources may end up in the food unintentionally, but these are also regulated as additives.

Grade the new safety rules. Originally, the FDA required companies to submit rigorous safety research to get a new additive approved. But for approval of common food ingredients, companies only needed to provide research that showed an ingredient was already Generally Recognized as Safe (GRAS). The FDA painstakingly reviewed the research for both GRAS and non-GRAS additives.

But in 1997, the FDA stopped requiring companies to submit research for GRAS products, settling for a research summary instead — and even that was optional. Many companies started submitting nearly all products as GRAS, including non-GRAS additives.

Some companies even declared their products as GRAS without seeking FDA approval. The Pew Charitable Trust estimates approximately 1,000 additives, labeled as GRAS, have been brought to market without being submitted for FDA approval.

Beware these additives. Experts say salt, sweeteners, and trans fats are the food additives you should worry about most, but you may also want to avoid these.

- Potassium bromate. Banned in other countries, this strengthens and stabilizes bread dough. It has been reduced or eliminated by most bakers.

- BHA (butylated hydroxyanisole) and BHT (butylated hydroxytoluene). Found in cereal, potato chips, gum, and oil, these chemicals prevent oils from becoming rancid, but they may also cause cancer.

- Nitrites and nitrates. These preservatives in packaged meats may help create cancer-causing compounds in your body.

- Sulfites. Found in vinegar, wine, packaged vegetables, and dried fruit, these preservatives may cause headaches or life-threatening reactions in some people with asthma.

- Monosodium glutamate (MSG). This flavor booster is added to many Chinese foods, frozen entrees, salad dressings, chips, dips, and soups. In large amounts, MSG may cause headaches, muscle aches, and flushing in some people.

- Caramel coloring. Some caramel coloring additives contain 4-methylimidazole (4-Mel), a suspected cancer-causer. Research by Consumer Reports suggests some caramel-colored soft drinks may not be safe, but you can't tell which ones. Some suggest avoiding all soft drinks.

- Artificial colors. These may cause allergic reactions in certain people, especially Yellow No. 5 or 6, Red No. 3 or 40, Blue No. 1 or 2, and Green No. 3.

These may not be the only additives to watch out for. Avoiding packaged, processed, and fast foods can help limit or eliminate other potentially unsafe additives.

If you need to avoid a specific food additive due to allergies or other health reasons, check ingredient labels carefully, but be aware that some items may not appear on food labels.

Visit *cspinet.org* for more information about individual additives.

Sweet nothings or health risk? The sour truth on artificial sugars

Artificial sweeteners won't cause cavities, raise your blood sugar, or add many calories to your diet. They're also super sweet, so you can use only a tiny amount. But some health watchdog groups are concerned about their safety, and the FDA has set Acceptable Daily Intake limits on how much you can consume daily without harm. Cut through the confusion, and make smarter choices with this quick guide to the most common artificial sweeteners.

Acesulfame potassium or acesulfame-K (Sunett, Sweet One).
Although the FDA has declared this safe, watchdog groups are
calling for new studies about possible thyroid damage and cancer
risk, and the Center for Science in the Public Interest (CSPI)
recommends you avoid it.

Aspartame (Equal, NutraSweet, Sugar Twin). Foods containing
aspartame also include the amino acid phenylalanine, so their
labels must include a statement about their phenylalanine content.
This helps people who have phenylketonuria — difficulty
digesting phenylalanine — avoid it.

Although the FDA declared aspartame safe, the CSPI recommends
avoiding it because of concerns about cancer. Some people also
report headaches and dizziness that may be related to aspartame.

Advantame. As the newest artificial sweetener approved by the
FDA, advantame needs time to develop established brand names.
Because advantame is a mix of vanillin and aspartame, it's much
sweeter than aspartame. So you need much less to reach your
preferred level of sweetness. Because the phenylalanine amounts
are so tiny, this sweetener doesn't require special labeling about
phenylalanine. Both the FDA and CSPI consider advantame safe.

Saccharin (Sweet'N Low, Sweet Twin). No longer considered a
cancer risk, the FDA has approved this sweetener as safe. Yet, the
CSPI recommends avoiding it, and some say a 150-pound person
should have no more than eight packets a day.

Sucralose (Splenda). Recent research suggests sucralose may cause
leukemia in mice exposed to the sweetener before birth. CSPI
recommends caution with this sweetener, but the FDA says it's safe.

When choosing and using artificial sweeteners, also remember
these important points.

- Equal Plus, Equal Original, Equal Spoonful, and some soft
  drinks contain two artificial sweeteners instead of one. Read

ingredient labels on all food and drink products to make sure you don't get an artificial sweetener you don't want.

- Most artificial sweeteners are available as tabletop sweeteners and can be used in baking, but aspartame can lose its sweetness at high temperatures. Only add it near the end of cooking.

Supermarket spotlight: Just say no to processed foods

"If it came from a plant, eat it; if it was made in a plant, don't." So says Michael Pollan, author of *The Omnivore's Dilemma*.

That's a lovely sentiment, but perhaps not so practical. Most items you buy in your supermarket, technically, come from a processing plant. They've been handled, washed, cut, and packaged — at the very least. But you'll learn there are degrees of processing. Hot dogs are processed, but then so is whole-wheat bread or a bag of spinach.

Avoid the worst offenders. In the best sense, processed foods are easy ways to get safe, complete nutrition. They are convenient time-savers that can have a long shelf life. In the worst sense, they are low in nutrients and high in calories; salt; sugar; refined flour; artificial flavorings, colorings, and sweeteners; and preservatives, like the nitrates in cured meats.

The following is not a scientific list. In fact, ask 10 different nutritionists and you'd probably get 10 very different lists. But these represent the type of processed foods you should avoid.

- soda
- hot dogs
- potato chips
- french fries
- snack cakes
- white bread
- candy bars
- cheese dips

What do they all have in common? They are heavily processed. Your first step toward better nutrition is to become smart on the levels of processing. The Academy of Nutrition and Dietetics explains them this way.

- Minimally processed foods, like cut vegetables and roasted nuts, are simply pre-prepped for convenience.

- Moderately processed foods, like canned tuna and most canned and frozen fruits and vegetables, make the most of their nutritional benefits while extending their shelf life.

- More heavily processed foods have ingredients added for flavor and texture, like sweeteners, spices, and oils, as well as colors and preservatives. Examples are jarred pasta sauce, salad dressing, yogurt, and ready-to-eat foods, like crackers, granola, and deli meat.

- The most heavily processed foods include frozen pizza and microwaveable dinners, as well as unhealthy snack foods like those in the list.

Strive for healthy habits. Here are some smart and easy ways to avoid processed foods.

- Shop only the perimeter of your grocery store, where you're more likely to find whole foods like meat, dairy, and produce.

- Make friends with your produce manager. Ask about seasonal fruits and vegetables, and the best way to select and prepare them. Learn about new or unusual produce you might not normally buy.

- Read ingredient lists and remember they are in descending order. The first few ingredients are those you'll be getting the most of.

- Shop at a farmers market.

- Learn how to decipher nutrition labels. This way you can eliminate items with too much salt, sugar, fat, and other unhealthy ingredients.

- Limit boxed and canned food items. Even those that seem harmless, like instant noodles, can be crammed with sodium and unhealthy saturated fat.

- Restrict your beverages to water, 100% juices, coffee, tea, and milk.

- Ban most fast food and all deep-fried foods.

- Make your own lunches.

- Whip up your own smoothies. Commercial ones have lots of added sugar. By blending your own, you control the calories.

Should science tinker with your food?

You've seen the phrase "Non-GMO" on food products. Or maybe you've heard your favorite vegetable is a genetically modified organism and wonder if it's a science experiment gone awry. Rest assured — it's not.

When a scientist tinkers with the DNA of a plant, animal, or insect, and inserts it into a food crop to improve it in some way, the altered plant is a genetically modified organism (GMO). One example is the vitamin-enriched tomato. Scientists created it by transferring a beta carotene gene from carrots into the cells of tomato leaves. The tomato, already ripe with nutrients, is now even more nourishing.

Another example is the Hawaiian papaya. In the early 1990s, a virus threatened to wipe out the tropical fruit, but scientists developed a virus-resistant crop. Today, 80% of Hawaii's papaya crop is genetically modified. Without this GMO plant, the Aloha State's papaya plantations would not have survived.

While both of these examples seem harmless, critics say GMOs can jeopardize your health. They believe scientists could create a crop that's resistant to antibiotics or triggers allergic reactions. But the Food and Drug Administration says there's no cause for concern, stating that GMOs undergo extensive evaluations and must meet the same requirements as normally bred plants.

As the debate continues, you can avoid or limit GMOs if you're uneasy about their long-term effects.

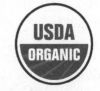

- Choose whole foods over processed since 70% of processed foods contain at least one GMO ingredient.

- If you buy processed foods, avoid items with corn or soy additives, which are more likely to be genetically modified.

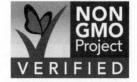

- Look for packages with the Non-GMO Project Verified seal or the USDA Organic seal.

3 meaty questions about going vegetarian

Vegetarian diets eliminate or restrict meats, including poultry and seafood, and may eliminate other animal products. Instead, meals focus on fruits, vegetables, whole grains, seeds, nuts, and legumes. There are several types of vegetarian diets.

- vegan — eliminates any food that comes from animals, including meats, fish, eggs, dairy products, and honey

- lacto-vegetarian — excludes meats, fish, and eggs, but allows dairy products

- flexitarian or semi-vegetarian — allows meat and fish occasionally

- ovo-vegetarian — eliminates meats, fish, and dairy products, but permits eggs

- pescetarian — excludes dairy products, eggs, and meats, but includes fish

Can it help with my health problems? Two studies suggest a vegan diet can mean lower cholesterol, more weight loss, and less medication for people with chronic diseases. This diet worked even better than the American Diabetes Association diet for people with diabetes.

Vegetarian diets may also help reduce blood pressure and blood sugar. What's more, vegetarian diets may help prevent cancer, obesity, cataracts, metabolic syndrome, and gallstones.

What pitfalls should I watch out for? You must still limit calories and fat, and avoid added oils, fats, and refined carbohydrates — both starches and sweets.

Also, eat a wide variety of foods to avoid nutritional deficiencies. Vegetarians may need to work harder to get enough iron, calcium, vitamin B12, protein, zinc, vitamin D, and omega-3 fatty acids. Eating fortified foods, like cereals and breads, or taking supplements can help, particularly for vitamins B12 and D. But also include foods like beans and nut butter for protein and iron, leafy greens and almonds for calcium, walnuts and flaxseed for omega-3 fatty acids, and white beans and pumpkin seeds for zinc.

Finally, eat combinations of proteins like grains and beans for complete proteins that include all the amino acids you need.

How can I get started? You can cut your food budget, make healthier meals, and keep your waistline slim — all with one versatile kitchen trick. Use inexpensive canned or dried beans in recipes instead of meat. Beans are rich in fiber, potassium, magnesium, folate, iron, lysine, and zinc. They're a good source of protein and resistant starch, a type of carbohydrate that won't make your blood sugar spike. Diets that include beans reduce LDL cholesterol and cut your risk of heart disease and diabetes. Beans may also help you feel full and control your weight.

Carbohydrates

Rev up your body with nature's energizers

Does the word carbohydrate conjure up pictures of apples, spinach, yogurt, or candy? Probably not. Most people don't realize these foods all contain carbohydrates. And just like the more well-known carbs in bread and pasta, they're your body's major source of energy. Cut out the carbs, and your body will suffer.

Carbohydrates get a bad rap because many people believe high-carb foods make you gain weight. But these super nutrients have important jobs like fueling your brain and central nervous system, keeping your digestive system regular, and providing the energy you need to keep your body moving. Jump on the low-carb bandwagon long enough, and you may end up feeling weak, dizzy, and constipated.

Even worse, when your body can't find carbohydrates for fuel, it will steal protein from your muscles for energy instead. When protein is broken down to make the sugar glucose, it can no longer be used to build muscle. That could lead to muscle weakness and kidney stress, along with other serious problems.

Understand the carb-energy connection. A carbohydrate is a compound made up of one or more sugar molecules. It's known as a macronutrient — along with protein and fat — because it's a major nutrient that supplies your body with calories, or energy.

Nutritionists divide carbohydrates into two groups — simple and complex — based on the number of molecules they have. You're probably familiar with some simple sugars like glucose, fructose, sucrose, and lactose. Starch and fiber are examples of complex carbohydrates.

Your body breaks down all carbohydrates into simple sugars, which the bloodstream absorbs. As your blood sugar levels rise, your pancreas releases a hormone called insulin to move the sugar from your blood into the cells, where it's used for energy.

The type of food you eat determines how quickly your blood sugar rises. For instance, when you bite into a food loaded with simple sugars like an apple or candy bar, your blood absorbs the sugars quickly, and your sugar levels spike. This sudden rise delivers a brief — but not lasting — burst of energy. Plus, you'll feel hungry again fairly soon. Complex carbs make your blood sugar rise slowly and steadily and deliver long-lasting fuel. That's because your body digests them before absorbing them into your bloodstream. Complex carbs also satisfy your hunger longer.

> Flip to the chapter *Probiotics* to learn how fiber feeds the healthy bacteria inside your body and helps in this powerful way to keep you happy and healthy.

Your body needs both types of energy for exercise. So here's a tip — before going for a walk, get a quick energy boost by drinking a cup of juice or eating a piece of toast with jelly. During a workout, munch on a handful of pretzels to keep going. Afterward, you need a light meal to restock your muscles with carbs. Try a granola bar or a bowl of cereal.

Pick carbs packed with nutrients. Bite into a plump peach, and you'll taste the sweetness of fructose. Nibble on a piece of chocolate, and your mouth will melt with the sugary sensation of sucrose. Both are delicious, but one gives you a burst of nutrition, and the other, mostly empty calories.

- Limit cakes and cookies that are full of sucrose or other added sugars. They provide few — if any — nutrients. An apple or banana loaded with natural fructose also delivers essential vitamins and minerals — a healthier choice.

- Choose whole grains over refined ones, and eat beans, peas, brown or wild rice, nuts and seeds, and vegetables with lots of fiber like broccoli and zucchini.

- Use the glycemic index (GI) — a chart that classifies foods depending on how quickly or slowly they raise your blood sugar. If you struggle with diabetes, the GI can help you make smart choices.

Know your daily needs. Eating the right amount of carbohydrates every day is as important as brushing your teeth. To meet your needs based on the Dietary Reference Intakes (DRI), try to get 45% to 65% of your calories from carbohydrates. That means if you eat around 2,000 calories a day, 900 to 1,300 of those calories should come from carbs. Or check packages for grams, and aim for 225 to 325 per day. Here's what a typical day might look like.

Carbohydrate foods	Grams	Calories
1 cup oatmeal	56	307
1 cup reduced-fat milk	12	122
2 slices whole-wheat toast	26	152
1 cup low-fat fruit yogurt	47	250
1 apple	25	95
1 banana	27	105
1 sweet potato	24	105
1/2 cup chocolate ice cream	19	143
Total	236	1,279

Without question, your body needs carbohydrates, so don't get swayed by popular opinion and cut these valuable nutrients out of your diet. Just make a point of eating nutrient-rich carbs. You'll reap tremendous health benefits, including the energy your brain and body need to get through each day.

Quick tip helps you ID healthy carbs

Some carbs, like fruits, vegetables, and whole grains, deliver an abundance of fiber and the nutrients your body needs for healthy living. They're also rich in important phytonutrients — plant chemicals that promote good health.

Others offer few to no nutrients. Manufacturers enrich some of these carbs with vitamins and minerals, but they can still contain too much fat, added sugar and salt, and preservatives. So how do you know which is which?

Your best bet is to read food labels and apply this simple formula created to help identify healthy whole-grain foods. Researchers at Harvard University have tested and endorsed it, but you don't have to be a math whiz to use it.

Step 1. Read the nutrition label and look for the amount of dietary fiber and total number of carbohydrates.

Step 2. Multiply the fiber by 10.

Step 3. If the result is equal to or greater than the total carbs, stock up — you've picked a nutrient-rich carb.

You can apply this formula to any food to determine if it's a "good" carb. Here's an example.

Step 1. A package of dried fruits and nuts — almonds, raisins, cherries, cranberries, and pistachios — contains 2 grams of dietary fiber and 16 grams of total carbs.

Step 2. 2 times 10 equals 20.

Step 3. 20 is higher than 16. This snack is a high-quality carb.

Don't be fooled by sneaky bread labels

No matter how you slice it, life without bread is no life at all. But how do you know which breads are best for you? The answer is easy — whole grains. Unfortunately, manufacturers like to put health claims like "all natural" and "multigrain" on bread bags. These claims can deceive if you don't know what to look for. Here's how to decipher which breads contain whole grains, and which ones don't.

- Make sure the nutrition label says 100% whole wheat or 100% whole grain as the first ingredient.

- Ignore packages with words like wheat, multigrain, seven-grain, and cracked wheat. Many manufacturers use these words to imply their breads are made with whole grains, but they're not.

- Look for the 100% whole-grain stamp. This seal, provided by the Whole Grains Council, a nonprofit that promotes the health benefits of whole grains, means all the bread's grain ingredients are whole grain. The stamp displays how many grams of whole grains are in each serving. To bear the stamp, the product must contain at least 16 grams per labeled serving, but it could have more, as seen in this example.

100% WHOLE GRAIN
23g or more per serving
WholeGrainsCouncil.org

100% OF THE GRAIN IS WHOLE GRAIN

- Learn to spot whole grains such as barley, buckwheat, millet, quinoa, whole oats, whole rye, and whole wheat.

- Put anything that says "unbleached" or "enriched" wheat flour back on the shelf. That's just another way of saying white flour.

- Don't buy a loaf of bread just because it's brown. The color doesn't mean it's whole wheat.

- Scan the list of ingredients for salt. Since most loaves of bread contain about 1 teaspoon of salt, and ingredients are listed in descending order by amount, any grain listed after salt would be insignificant.

Now it's time to test your knowledge. Can you pick out the healthiest bread from the two ingredient lists?

Multigrain bread	Whole-wheat bread
Unbleached Enriched Wheat Flour, Water, Wheat Gluten, Cellulose, Yeast, Soybean Oil, Honey, **Salt**, Barley, Natural Flavor Preservatives, Monocalcium Phosphate, Millet, Corn, Oats, Soybean Flour, Brown Rice, Flaxseed	100% Whole-Grain Whole-Wheat Flour, Water, Oat Fiber, Wheat Gluten, Yeast, Brown Sugar, Contains 2% Or Less Of The Following: **Salt**, Dough Conditioners, Fumaric Acid, Yeast Nutrients, Flaxseed, Wheat Starch, Calcium Propionate, Potassium Sorbate, Natamycin And Gamma Cyclodextrin, Soy Lecithin

If you picked the whole-wheat bread, give yourself an A+. This loaf contains 100% whole wheat. The multigrain bread lists unbleached enriched wheat flour as its first ingredient. This is not a whole grain. And the label mentions barley, millet, corn, oats, and brown rice after salt, so this bread includes minimal amounts of those grains.

5 reasons to give fiber a high-five

You want your digestive system to run as smoothly as a well-oiled machine. Only fiber can do that. It's the secret weapon that supercharges your digestive health.

Your body cannot digest fiber. This gives it a chance to slide through your digestive tract, slowing down or speeding up digestion. The speed of digestion depends on which type of fiber you're eating — soluble or insoluble.

- Soluble fiber absorbs water like a sponge, but turns into a gel as it slowly glides through your gut. Beans, nuts, berries, and oatmeal pack powerful amounts of soluble fiber.

- Insoluble fiber bulks up and softens your stool and helps it sail through your intestines. When you eat barley, brown rice, whole-grain cereals, and some fruits and vegetables with their skins, you're getting insoluble fiber.

6 surprisingly tasty sources of fiber

If you think fiber tastes like cardboard, you're in for a surprise. These treats will tickle your taste buds while serving up a healthy dose of fiber.

- Grapefruit. Skip the juice and go straight for the fruit. This citrus sweetheart packs fiber in a gel-like substance called pectin.

- Olives. Toss these in a salad or pasta dish for a savory source of fiber.

- Artichoke hearts. Saute in a little bit of olive oil with garlic, and add to a casserole to boost fiber without a lot of calories.

- Hazelnuts. Go nuts over this fabulous source of fiber. Half a cup serves up about 6 grams. Toss them into a fruit salad for a crunchy treat.

- Dark chocolate. Let a 1.4-ounce serving melt in your mouth, and you'll enjoy a jumbo serving of fiber — about 3 to 6 grams.

- Raspberries. Enjoy a cup of raspberries for a whopping 8 grams of fiber. They taste great over plain yogurt or a bowl of whole-grain cereal.

Most fruits and vegetables deliver a one-two punch, providing both kinds of fiber. For instance, a pear has over 2 grams of soluble fiber and almost 4 grams of insoluble fiber. And a half cup of sweet potatoes boasts almost 2 grams of soluble fiber and over 2 grams of insoluble.

Eating both types of fiber daily fights all sorts of digestive distress. Here's a look at what sensational fiber can do for you.

Conquers constipation. Everyone's bowel habits are different, but many doctors say you're constipated if you go to the bathroom less than three times a week. And while constipation can mean you're not drinking enough water or getting enough exercise, it could just mean you're not getting enough fiber. Try drinking plenty of water and eating insoluble fiber like fruits, veggies, or whole grains.

Defeats diarrhea. Bacteria, parasites, viruses, even some medications can keep you running to the bathroom. To treat mild to moderate cases, try soluble fiber like oatmeal, bananas, and mashed potatoes. These foods will soak up water from your intestines and firm up your stool.

> If you're not used to eating a lot of fiber, add it gradually and drink plenty of liquids. Too much fiber can make you feel gassy, crampy, and bloated. Follow the *Dietary Guidelines for Americans*, which recommends a daily total of 25 grams for women and 38 grams for men.

Guards against gallstones. Many people go through life with gallstones and don't know it. But some suffer severe pain, fever, chills, and vomiting. Gallstones form when bile salts containing cholesterol crystallize. Their sizes range from a grain of sand to a golf ball. These stones can block the passage between your gallbladder and your liver.

Soluble fiber soaks up bile salts and flushes them out of your system. Insoluble fiber carries food through your gut quickly, so bile doesn't have time to form stones in your gallbladder.

Beware hidden supplement dangers

Fiber supplements, including the herb psyllium, could interfere with the absorption of medications you take and minerals you need. Fiber sweeps them through your digestive system without giving your body time to use them.

- Medications. If you are on drugs for your heart, to lower cholesterol, or to control diabetes, experts suggest taking fiber supplements two to three hours before or after you take your medications. These include popular prescriptions like Crestor, Plavix, and Lipitor.

- Minerals. Your body needs iron, zinc, calcium, and magnesium for good health. But excess fiber in your diet can bind with these minerals and flush them out too quickly. Stick to the recommended daily allowance of fiber and you shouldn't have a problem.

Soothes irritable bowel syndrome. If you suffer from frequent bouts of diarrhea and constipation, plus bloating, nausea, and headaches, you may have irritable bowel syndrome (IBS). No one really knows why people develop IBS, but some doctors believe stress or foods that produce gas play a role. Relieve symptoms with foods high in soluble fiber — apples, strawberries, oats, nuts, and seeds. Stay away from high-fiber wheat bran. It could make IBS worse.

Calms ulcers. Although the bacterium *H. pylori* causes most ulcers, you're also at risk if you take nonsteroidal anti-inflammatory drugs (NSAIDs), like ibuprofen and aspirin, for arthritis. These painful sores usually affect the stomach or the first part of your small intestine. Some studies show eating high-fiber foods lowers your risk of getting ulcers. Soluble fibers seem to lessen the amount of stomach acid your body makes, which can help ulcers heal.

Short-circuit those sugar cravings

Most Americans get about 30 teaspoons of added sugar every day. That's a whopping 228 cups a year. And extra pounds aren't the only problem with added sugar. Your chances of dying from heart disease go way up when you guzzle too much of the sweet stuff. In fact, in a recent study, the risk jumped 38% for people who got 17% to 21% of their calories from added sugar compared to those who got just 8%.

Other studies show added sugar may raise blood pressure, triglyceride levels, and LDL cholesterol, and contribute to inflammation — all key factors in heart disease. Bitter news if you have a sweet tooth.

Thankfully, you don't have to give up sweet treats completely to maintain good health. You just need to know your limits. Keep these suggestions in mind the next time you crave something sweet.

Know how low you should go. No one likes to count grams and calories — especially for sweets. But if you want to live healthy, you need to know how much sugar is too much. Look at the table below with recommendations from the *Dietary Guidelines for Americans*.

If you eat this many calories a day, don't eat or drink more than this much added sugar.

1,600 calories	4 teaspoons or about 16 grams
1,800 calories	5 teaspoons or about 20 grams
2,000 to 2,200 calories	8 teaspoons or about 32 grams
2,400 calories	10 teaspoons or 40 grams

To put things in perspective, think about this. A 12-ounce can of soda contains around 38 grams of sugar. That's more than 8 teaspoons — too much sugar for one day if you eat around 2,000 calories.

Solve the secret to sugar names. Added sugars parade across food labels with sneaky names. Here's an easy way to find them. If a word ends in -ose, like maltose or sucrose, it's an added sugar.

Other added sugars end with the words "syrup," like corn syrup, or "concentrate," as in fruit juice concentrate.

But remember, new food labels will show the amount of added sugars in grams.

Sweet ways to swap out sugar. As you cut back on sugar, you may need a few ideas to get you through the day. Here's a list to get you started.

- Sweeten bland foods like oatmeal with spices. Try cloves, nutmeg, cinnamon, or allspice.

- Slash the amount of sugar you use in recipes by up to a third without changing the taste.

- Swap out the sugar in baked goods with almond, lemon, orange, or vanilla extract.

- Instead of popping candies or cookies, pair a banana or berries with a small piece of dark chocolate for a sweet but nutritious treat.

- Eat regular meals that combine protein, whole grains, fruits, and vegetables throughout your day. This will keep your blood sugar stable and cut out cravings for sweets.

High fructose corn syrup: One spoonful of trouble

Gulp down a sugary soda, and your taste buds explode with the sweetness of high fructose corn syrup (HFCS). Many critics believe HFCS is harmful — more harmful than other added sugars. But others say it's no better or worse.

This popular sweetener is a combination of two simple sugars — fructose and glucose. Because HFCS tastes sweeter than regular sugar, manufacturers can use less, which saves them money. You'll find HFCS in everything from soda to pancake syrup. Scientists spend a lot of time studying HFCS, and what they're learning may surprise you.

- Too much high fructose corn syrup can lead to weight gain and more belly fat, Princeton University researchers found during an animal study. That's a concern because those conditions can trigger heart disease and diabetes.

- More people suffer from type 2 diabetes in countries that use a lot of HFCS than countries that don't. Researchers from the University of Southern California, after comparing data from 43 countries, made this interesting discovery.

- On the other hand, a team of researchers recently debunked the theory that large amounts of high fructose corn syrup contributes to nonalcoholic fatty liver disease. After reviewing studies, they found no link between the two, according to their article published in the *American Journal of Clinical Nutrition*.

While research over high fructose corn syrup continues, many experts say the real issue is not the added sugar itself — it's people's obsession with all added sugars. They just can't get enough. And that in itself causes problems.

For example, people who drink sodas don't feel as full as people who get the same number of calories from food, so they tend to eat just as much as if they hadn't guzzled a soft drink, according to a Harvard School of Public Health study. It's not necessarily the HFCS — it's that soft drinks don't fill you up like other carbs.

This tendency to overeat is a major problem, says Dr. John Sievenpiper, a researcher at St. Michael's Hospital in Toronto.

"The debate over the role of fructose in obesity, fatty liver, and other metabolic diseases has distracted us from the issue of overconsumption," he says. "Our data should serve to remind people that the excess calories, whether they are from fructose or other sources, are the issue."

The message is clear — no matter what type of added sugar you are talking about, cut back.

Fats

5 fabulous fat facts you need to know

Fat is not just the jiggly stuff around your belly and thighs. It's a nutrient every person needs to stay healthy. Surprised? Most people are, considering "fat" is like a four-letter word today. But as you learn more about nutrition, you'll realize fat is something you can't live without.

You need a certain amount of good dietary fats to stay healthy. These pour on the benefits without packing on inches or wreaking havoc in your arteries. In fact, the good fats found in nuts, plants, and fish deliver a slew of benefits to your body.

- When you exercise, you use carbs for energy for the first 20 minutes. But then it's the calories from fat that give you the power you need to keep going.

- Your body can't absorb vitamins A, D, E, and K without fat. That's why they're called fat-soluble vitamins.

- Fats make foods flavorful and help you feel full.

- Certain cells in your body need fats to help keep you warm.

- Your hair and skin need fats to stay strong and healthy.

The surprising truth about good-for-you fats

Beware — fats are not created equal. There are three types, and while each may pack the same amount of calories per gram, they are very different when it comes to your health.

Saturated fats spell trouble for your heart. Think butter, shortening, and the white marbled fat in meat — all of these are solid at room temperature. And they're loaded with saturated fat, which can trigger life-threatening heart disease and the blood clotting associated with heart attacks.

Limit these by eating no more than 22 grams of saturated fat a day, based on a 2,000-calorie diet.

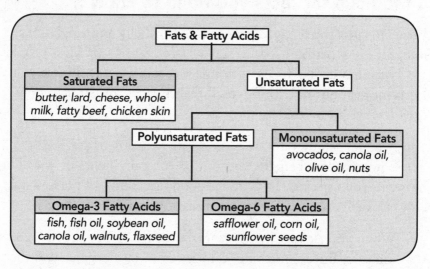

Polyunsaturated fatty acids (PUFAs) must be in balance.
You've probably heard of omega-3 fatty acids, the polyunsaturated fats found in fish like salmon, tuna, and halibut. But you may not know your body can't make omega-3. So you must get it through your diet. Research shows this fat helps prevent cancer and heart disease, reduces inflammation, and keeps your mind and memory sharp.

A distant cousin to omega-3 is omega-6 fatty acid. They're similar in that your body can't make omega-6 either, so you have to get it from food. Studies show omega-6 promotes brain function, lowers blood pressure, and reduces your risk of diabetes.

The key to getting the greatest health benefits from these two fatty acids is balance. Omega-3s seem to reduce inflammation, while some omega-6 fatty acids promote it. The ideal ratio of omega-6 to omega-3 is 4 to 1, but the typical American diet is closer to 20 to 1.

Eating more fish, fresh fruits and vegetables, whole grains, garlic, and olive oil — and less meat — can help you achieve a healthy balance. These food choices are typical of the Mediterranean Diet.

Monounsaturated fatty acids (MUFAs) are essential. This type of fat is found in a variety of foods and oils, including nuts like macadamias and hazelnuts, and oils like olive and safflower. Studies show eating foods rich in MUFAs may control insulin and blood sugar levels, which is especially helpful for people with type 2 diabetes. In addition MUFAs can help prevent arthritis, high blood pressure, and even cancer.

Easy ways to boost your good fats. Choose fats wisely to reap the benefits. Experts recommend you get 20% to 35% of your daily total calories from fats, primarily unsaturated fats. Here's a list of ideas to get you started.

- Bake, grill, broil, or steam foods instead of frying.

- Trade meat for seafood like salmon or mackerel twice a week. Stick with a 4-ounce serving.

- Pick fat-free or low-fat cheese, milk, and ice cream over those loaded with fat.

- Use olive oil to make marinades and salad dressings, and to saute vegetables.

- Add flavor to your foods with herbs, lemon juice, salsa, or vinegar instead of with butter and cream-based sauces.

- Steer clear of solid fats like lard and butter. Go with olive or canola oil, or a margarine that lists liquid vegetable oil as its first ingredient.

- Trim the skin from chicken and excess fat from steaks before cooking.

- Look for the number of fat grams on Nutrition Facts labels when you shop for groceries.

Does low-fat dieting harm your heart?

Low-fat diets can create chaos in your body, including weight gain. Before you jump on the low-fat bandwagon, get the latest facts.

- Food manufacturers pour added sugar into low-fat foods to make them taste better. The label may say low-fat, but the calories can be through the roof. What's more, these foods raise your blood triglycerides and lower your good HDL cholesterol — a dangerous combo for your heart.

- Low-fat diets exclude foods like nuts, seeds, fish, and vegetable oils, which are bursting with nutrients. So you don't get the vitamins, minerals, and phytochemicals you need for a healthy heart.

- Research shows low-fat diets may lower bad cholesterol, but not the risk of dying from heart disease.

- Several studies from the Women's Health Initiative suggest that older women eating low-fat diets did not lower their risk for stroke, heart disease, breast cancer, or colon cancer. The study followed postmenopausal women for over eight years.

While more research needs to be done, experts recommend you add some healthy fats to your daily diet.

Omega-3 fatty acids: Essential nutrients that pack a mega punch

Your body can't make omega-3 fatty acids, but you can get this amazing nutrient from salmon and other fish, which are rich in two kinds — docosahexaenoic acid (DHA) and eicosapentaenoic acid (EPA). These battle inflammation, which scientists say may be the root of many chronic conditions like high blood pressure, cancer, depression, diabetes, and arthritis.

Experts believe omega-3s work by blocking two of your body's chemicals — cytokines and prostaglandins — that trigger inflammation. They also pump up your body's anti-inflammatory chemicals called resolvins. This one-two punch can knock out all sorts of health problems.

Soothe achy joints. Several studies show that omega-3s from fish can ease morning stiffness and lessen the need for nonsteroidal anti-inflammatory drugs (NSAIDs).

Preserve your memories. Researchers at Columbia University found that eating fish can fend off dementia in people with mild memory loss.

Keep your ticker ticking. People who eat more than two servings of fish a week show less atherosclerosis in their carotid artery than those who eat little to none.

Shake off blood sugar problems. A study from the Center for Genetics, Nutrition, and Health shows a diet rich in omega-3 fatty acids from seafood curbs the harmful effects of a diet high in sugar.

Now that you know the health benefits of omega-3s, you'll want to go fishing for good sources. Make sure you add the following foods to your shopping list.

- walnuts
- canola oil
- flaxseed and flaxseed oil
- fatty fish, like salmon, mackerel, herring, and tuna

Beware the hidden dangers in trans fats

Trans fats spell trouble. They raise your bad LDL cholesterol and lower your good HDL cholesterol, increasing your risk of heart disease. That's why the Food and Drug Administration is banning them.

This unhealthy fat is produced during a process called hydrogenation, when hydrogen is added to polyunsaturated oil so it remains solid at room temperature. The oil becomes more stable and helps foods stay fresher longer. It's most commonly found in shortening, margarine, snack foods, store-bought baked goods, and fried foods in restaurants.

Many health experts believe lowering the amount of trans fats in the American diet could prevent 20,000 heart attacks and 7,000 deaths from heart disease a year. But many bakers disagree. They believe trans fats in trace amounts are not harmful and are a critical ingredient in many baked goods.

Although the Food and Drug Administration has declared war on trans fat and is working to require food makers to gradually phase out its use, you can still find it in many products. Avoid packages with the words "trans fat" or "partially hydrogenated oils" and dodge the danger completely by eating whole, fresh foods instead of prepackaged ones.

Fish oil supplements: OK or no way?

Not a fish lover? You're not alone. If you want to add omega-3s to your diet, consider taking supplements — with caution.

Studies show fish oil supplements may reduce the inflammation that can lead to heart disease, diabetes, and memory loss. Combine them with aspirin, and you get a double whammy. Researchers from Brigham and Women's Hospital and Harvard Medical School found that when you take aspirin with fish oil supplements, they work together even better to combat inflammation.

Before you try this combo, talk with your doctor. Fish oil supplements and aspirin can have serious side effects, like thinning your blood. You shouldn't take them if you already take a blood thinner, such as Coumadin (warfarin).

Protein

Power up with the essential bodybuilder

Protein is one nutrient your body absolutely needs to function. It's in every cell in your body, and no other nutrient plays as many different roles in keeping you alive and healthy. Protein's most important job is to build and repair tissue, but it also has other crucial roles.

- provides the enzymes and hormones you need for metabolism, digestion, and other critical processes

- maintains your body's fluid balance

- carries nutrients throughout your body

- helps your immune system fight infection and your blood clot properly

Your body creates this amazing nutrient from 20 building blocks called amino acids. Nine of these are essential amino acids, which means you must get them from food. The others are nonessential. You still need them, but your body can make them, so you don't have to get them from other sources. Your body can't store protein like it does fat and carbohydrates, so you need a new supply of amino acids every day.

Choose your sources wisely. Animal-based products like beef, poultry, fish, milk, cheese, and eggs are the top sources because they contain all the essential amino acids. They are known as complete, or high-quality, proteins. Some crops, like soybeans and quinoa, are complete proteins, but most plants are incomplete because they don't have all the amino acids. Nuts, seeds, beans, grains, and vegetables are examples of incomplete proteins.

If plant foods are already the mainstay of your diet, you don't have to worry. Simply combine incomplete proteins to get the full range of amino acids your body needs. Rice and beans is a typical combination that does the job. Or take a cue from your childhood, and eat a peanut butter sandwich. You don't have to eat the complementary proteins in the same meal — just make sure it's the same day.

Your perfect protein plan. Because protein is such a critical nutrient, you need to make sure you get enough each day. The Recommended Dietary Allowance (RDA) is 46 grams (g) for adult women and 56 g for men. But your body needs to replace protein tissue every day, so larger people actually have a higher protein need than those who weigh less. To figure out what's right for you, multiply 0.36 grams for each pound of body weight. If you weigh 140 pounds, you'll find you need 50 g of protein to meet your daily requirements.

But don't overdo it — for the average 140-pound person, more than 125 grams a day would probably be too much, say experts at Harvard. An overload of protein can strain your liver and kidneys and make it more difficult for your body to absorb other nutrients. Plus eating lots of meat can overload your body with saturated fat and cholesterol. A 9-ounce T-bone steak, for example, contains a whopping 62 g of protein, 20 g of saturated fat, and 168 milligrams of cholesterol. Look for healthy protein choices like low-fat milk and yogurt or fat-free cheese.

Experts recommend you include protein-rich foods at each meal to reap the most benefit. To get a balanced supply throughout the day, choose foods like these.

- 1 cup oatmeal 6 g
- 8 oz Greek yogurt 17 g
- 3 oz beef or poultry 25 g
- 1 cup edamame 17 g
- 1 oz almonds 6 g
- 1 cup low-fat milk 8 g
- 1 egg 6 g
- 1 cup quinoa 8 g
- 1/2 cup black beans 7 g
- 1 oz pumpkin seeds 5 g

The beef with red meat: Simple swap may save your life

It doesn't seem to matter whether you smoke or drink alcohol, how much you exercise, or even how old you are. If you eat red meat, especially processed meat like bacon, sausage, and hot dogs, experts say you are putting your health — and your life — at risk.

While most people think of red meat as an important source of protein, they forget it's high in saturated fat, a type of dietary fat that raises the amount of cholesterol in your blood. In addition, highly processed meats give you a whopping dose of salt, preservatives, and substances known to increase the risk of cancer.

A new study, published in the leading medical journal *The BMJ*, analyzed data from more than 80,000 participants in the Nurses' Health Study and the Health Professionals Follow-up Study. They found, to reduce your risk of diabetes, heart disease, cancer, COPD, and high blood pressure, it's not enough to simply cut back on the bacon. You must replace red meat with nuts, fish, dairy, eggs, legumes, and other healthy sources of protein.

Preserve your pizzazz with protein

You can stay active no matter what your age, plus help your body ward off disease, by simply getting the right amount of protein each day. This easy addition to your diet plan may be just what your body needs.

Research shows that up to 24% of older women are protein deficient because they're eating fewer protein-rich foods. To make matters worse, the older you get, the harder it is for your body to absorb and process protein. That means it's struggling to build and maintain your cells and tissues without the critical building blocks it needs. Add more protein to your diet, and you'll give your body a fighting chance. Here are some ways it can help.

Maintains muscle strength. You naturally lose muscle mass as you age, but losing muscle strength and function leads to a serious condition known as sarcopenia. Physical activity, particularly strength training, is the best way to prevent this condition. Research also suggests older adults can combat muscle decline by eating more protein. A seven-year study of 5,000 postmenopausal women found that those who included more protein in their diets functioned better physically than those who got the fewest calories from protein.

Supports your heart. Remember, your heart is a muscle, and protein helps build muscle. But you need to get the right kind of protein to strengthen your heart and fight off disease. Research shows that eating protein-rich foods like nuts, fish, poultry, and low-fat dairy significantly lowers your risk of heart disease compared with eating red meat, processed meats, and high-fat dairy.

Battles osteoporosis. Experts used to think excess protein hurt bone density by leaching out calcium. Instead, recent research suggests protein may work with calcium to prevent bone loss. In one study, scientists found that older women's bones may benefit from more protein, especially if their calcium levels are low. Another study showed that supplementing with the amino acids phenylalanine, tyrosine, and tryptophan helped increase bone mass in older animals.

Balances blood sugar levels. Adding protein to your morning meal could be just the thing to even out your glucose levels and lower your risk of developing diabetes. And if you have type 2 diabetes, studies show that including protein and healthy fat in a hearty breakfast may help you control blood sugar as well as hunger.

Although the RDA for adult women is 46 grams, don't be afraid to eat more. New research from Purdue University suggests older women would benefit from eating 29% more protein than recommended daily, or about 59 grams.

"Our data suggests that the current dietary protein requirement estimate may be too low and reinforces that more research is needed to identify accurate protein amounts for older adults," says nutrition science professor Wayne W. Campbell, an expert on dietary protein and human health. "These findings, along with previous research, indicate that consuming amounts of protein moderately above the current RDA may be helpful."

Delicious food fix for thinning hair

Want to grow stronger, thicker hair? One natural beauty staple will help you do just that — eggs.

Perhaps you've used eggs as a conditioning hair mask that you wash out in the shower. Folk wisdom says to apply whole eggs for normal hair, egg yolks for dry hair, and egg whites for oily hair. But eating this delicious source of protein also supplies your hair with the nutrients it needs, from the inside out.

As you age, your hair may naturally thin, losing volume and thickness — perhaps because the follicles stop producing hair, or because your hair shafts become finer.

Let eggs come to the rescue. Besides protein, eggs contain the B vitamin biotin. Both help strengthen your hair follicles, boost hair growth, and keep your hair supple and shiny.

Vitamins

Revitalize your life with vitamins

In Latin, "vita" means life and "amines" means organic substances. Put the two together and what do you get? Vitamins — organic nutrients that are vital to life.

A healthy diet filled with fruits, vegetables, and whole grains provides all the vitamins you need — 13 in fact. You need these vitamins for your body to grow and digest food. Your nerves also need them to work properly.

Like actors in a movie, each vitamin plays a leading role or supporting role in your body. For example, you need vitamin A to help you see better, especially at night. Vitamin D helps you absorb calcium for healthy bones.

Nutritionists divide vitamins into two groups — fat-soluble and water-soluble.

- Vitamins A, D, E, and K are fat-soluble. This simply means your fat cells store them, and your body can hang on to them for weeks, even months. When they're needed, special protein carriers ferry them through your blood.

- The B vitamins and vitamin C are water-soluble. Your body absorbs them quickly and gets rid of any extra in your urine.

It's best to get vitamins from the foods you eat, but people on restrictive diets may need to take supplements. Check with your doctor first.

Read on to learn more about these life-giving nutrients and find out how many grams (g), milligrams (mg), or micrograms (mcg) you need each day.

Vitamins and minerals: How much is enough?

Learning how much of each nutrient you need daily can seem like rocket science. And in many ways, it is a science. But it's an easy one to digest with the help of Dietary Reference Intakes, or DRIs.

Established by a group of researchers in the United States and Canada, DRIs include Recommended Dietary Allowances (RDAs) and Adequate Intakes (AIs) for almost every nutrient imaginable.

RDA levels are based on scientific research. They tell you how much of a nutrient most healthy people of a particular age group and gender should get each day. AIs are set when scientists have too little data to establish an RDA value.

As you learn more about DRIs, remember that these numbers are the recommended — not required — safe amounts for people in each age and gender group.

Fat-soluble vitamins

Vitamin A. This was the first fat-soluble vitamin to be discovered, earning it the honor of the first letter of the alphabet for its name. Your body needs vitamin A for many important functions. Your eyesight depends on an adequate supply of vitamin A. It is also needed by your epithelial tissues, which include your skin and the internal linings of your body. Vitamin A assists in bone growth and it helps keep your immune system healthy, so you can fight off infections.

One sweet potato, half a cup of cooked spinach, and half a cup of raw carrots each contain more than the amount you need daily.

Vitamin A	DRI women	age 51+	700 mcg
	DRI men	age 51+	900 mcg

Vitamin D. Why do people call this one the sunshine vitamin? Because your body makes vitamin D when your skin is kissed by the sun. You can also get a heap of D from foods like tuna, sardines, and fortified yogurt and milk. Get your daily dose by serving up 3 ounces of salmon for dinner. You'll be glad you did because vitamin D helps your body absorb calcium and phosphorus — two nutrients that keep your skeleton strong.

Vitamin D			
	DRI women	age 51-70	15 mcg or 600 IU
		age 71+	20 mcg or 800 IU
	DRI men	age 51-70	15 mcg or 600 IU
		age 71+	20 mcg or 800 IU

Vitamin E. Breathing is a dangerous proposition without this fat-soluble vitamin. Natural actions like this produce free radicals — unstable compounds that attack your body's cells and nutrients. In the process, they produce more free radicals, starting a chain reaction that can lead to cancer, heart disease, and other chronic illnesses. Vitamin E stops this snowball before it starts rolling.

Your body also needs vitamin E to boost your immune system, help widen blood vessels, and keep blood from clotting.

Nuts and seeds are well-known sources of vitamin E. You'll also find it in wheat germ, green vegetables, fortified cereals and juices, whole grains, and vegetable oils.

Vitamin E			
	DRI women	age 51+	15 mg
	DRI men	age 51+	15 mg

Vitamin K. This vitamin isn't on any food's nutrition label, but it's still important. Without vitamin K, your blood couldn't clot. It also helps your body use calcium and ensures that your bones stay strong. Vitamin K compounds include K1, which is the main dietary form, and K2, which is present in small amounts in certain animal-based and fermented foods. K2 compounds are also produced by bacteria in your gut.

Green vegetables like spinach, kale, broccoli, turnip and mustard greens, collards, and Swiss chard are the primary sources of vitamin K1. Don't overdo them if you're on blood thinners like warfarin, as vitamin K can decrease the effects of the medicine.

Vitamin K	DRI women	age 51+	90 mcg
	DRI men	age 51+	120 mcg

Water-soluble vitamins

Biotin. Also known as vitamin B7, this B-complex vitamin assists in the release of energy from carbohydrates, fats, and proteins so you can have more energy and feel healthier. It's also a boon to your hair and nails. Biotin is found naturally in meat, milk, almonds, sunflower seeds, and even some vegetables, including Swiss chard and sweet potatoes. One egg contains 10 micrograms (mcg) of biotin, and you'll get 5 mcg from a delicious 3-ounce serving of salmon.

Biotin	DRI women	age 51+	30 mcg
	DRI men	age 51+	30 mcg

Folate. This is one heart-saving, brain-boosting, stroke-stopping, mood-enhancing B vitamin you shouldn't miss out on. First of all, you need it to manufacture DNA that is essential to creating new cells all over your body. But it does so much more, like lowering the level of artery-damaging homocysteine in your body that contributes to heart disease and stroke. Research has shown folate-rich foods may also help ward off depression and memory loss.

The name comes from a Latin word meaning "leaf," so as you might expect, it's naturally found in green leafy vegetables like spinach and mustard greens. You'll also get your fill of folate from asparagus, Brussels sprouts, and legumes. You'll find a form of folate, called folic acid, in fortified foods and dietary supplements.

Folate	DRI women	age 51+	400 mcg
	DRI men	age 51+	400 mcg

Niacin. Like the other B vitamins, vitamin B3 helps your body change carbohydrates into sugar for fuel. That means it plays a big role in cranking up your energy. Think of vitamin B3, or niacin, like a car's engine. The food you eat is the gas that makes the car (your body) run. But you need something to help convert that gas into mechanical power. Niacin sets off the chemical reactions that transform food into the energy that keeps you going.

Plus this nutrient is so powerful it also helps increase blood flow, manage your cholesterol, and fortify your mind.

You can get about half of your daily amount by eating a 3-ounce serving of either grilled chicken breast or roasted turkey breast. Niacin is also plentiful in plant-based foods like brown rice, marinara sauce, and tuna.

Niacin	DRI women	age 51+	14 mg
	DRI men	age 51+	16 mg

Pantothenic acid. This nutrient, also called vitamin B5, helps turn the food you eat into the energy you need to make the most of your day. It's especially important for creating and breaking down fats in your body.

Pantothenic acid gets its name from the Greek word that means "from all sides." That makes sense because experts say most plant- and animal-based foods contain this vitamin in varying amounts. Some of the richest sources are beef, chicken, whole grains, and vegetables like mushrooms, avocados, and broccoli. Many breakfast cereals are fortified with 100% of your daily B5 needs.

Pantothenic acid	DRI women	age 51+	5 mg
	DRI men	age 51+	5 mg

Riboflavin. Vitamin B2, another name for this nutrient, is a real team player. It works with the other B vitamins to provide you with energy and healthy skin and eyes, and it may help your body absorb iron better. People who have low iron often have low levels of riboflavin, too. Riboflavin also helps your adrenal glands produce hormones.

To get your daily dose of riboflavin, eat a variety of foods like almonds, quinoa, and low-fat yogurt. One cup of cooked spinach gets you a quarter of the recommended daily amount.

Riboflavin	DRI women	age 51+	1.1 mg
	DRI men	age 51+	1.3 mg

Thiamine. To process energy, every cell in your body needs thiamine (vitamin B1). It also plays important roles in the function of your nerves, muscles, and heart. You need thiamine for your nerves to carry signals from your brain to other parts of your body, so it helps keep your brain and your body working efficiently.

Whole grains, pork, fish, and legumes are all good sources of thiamine. A cup of black beans boasts 33% of your daily needs.

Thiamine	DRI women	age 51+	1.1 mg
	DRI men	age 51+	1.2 mg

Vitamin B6. This water-soluble vitamin, also known as pyridoxine, plays a role in developing your brain and keeping your nervous and immune systems healthy. Low levels of B6 have been associated with symptoms of depression.

Research has found that vitamin B6 works with folate and vitamin B12 to control high levels of homocysteine in your blood. This common amino acid can damage your arteries, making it a risk factor for heart disease.

Vitamin B6 is naturally present in many foods. A baked potato, 3-ounce chicken breast, and an avocado provide all the vitamin B6 you need for a day. Other good sources include chickpeas, spinach, salmon, tuna, beef, turkey, bananas, and sweet potatoes.

| **Vitamin B6** | DRI women | age 51+ | 1.5 mg |
| | DRI men | age 51+ | 1.7 mg |

Vitamin B12. This nutrient could win an MVP award for all the ways it helps you stay healthy. It keeps your nerve and blood cells strong, helps make DNA, and prevents megaloblastic anemia, which makes people tired and weak.

To make sure you get enough vitamin B12 in your diet, eat chicken liver or sardines, sirloin steak, tuna packed in water, and cottage cheese. Amazingly, 3 ounces of cooked clams contain 1,402% of your daily needs.

Unfortunately, up to 15% of older adults are deficient in this important B vitamin because they no longer have enough stomach acid to help absorb the natural form of B12 from food. The good news is those folks can still absorb some of the synthetic B12 in supplements and fortified foods like cereal.

| **Vitamin B12** | DRI women | age 51+ | 2.4 mg |
| | DRI men | age 51+ | 2.4 mg |

Vitamin C. This is probably the most famous vitamin of all, renown as a cold cure, a cancer fighter, and the king of antioxidants. Vitamin C deserves all the attention. It safeguards you from free radicals, and it's also in charge of making collagen. This substance

ligaments, tendons, and scar tissue. It also supports your bones and teeth.

Citrus fruits like oranges and grapefruit may be the first foods that come to mind when you think of vitamin C. But you can also find it in other fruits and veggies such as broccoli, Brussels sprouts, strawberries, and kiwi. Eat half a cup of raw sweet red peppers to score 106% of the amount your body needs each day.

Vitamin C	DRI women	age 51+	75 mg
	DRI men	age 51+	90 mg

5 vitamin myths you shouldn't believe

Americans shell out a whopping $5 billion in vitamin supplements every year. That's big business for supplement suppliers. And who wouldn't want to take a multivitamin? Their labels make them sound like you can't live without them. But are supplements all they're cracked up to be?

Take, for example, one popular multivitamin that claims it can lower your risk of heart disease. Research shows multivitamins can do no such thing. To be a savvy health consumer, you need to separate fact from fiction.

Antioxidant vitamins prevent cancer. You've heard this popular myth for decades. But study after study has shown taking antioxidant supplements do nothing to prevent or battle cancer. One alarming piece of research published in the *Annals of Internal Medicine* suggests beta carotene supplements actually raise the risk of lung cancer in people at high risk, like smokers.

A review of 14 trials found the supplements A, C, E, and beta carotene, which were taken to prevent intestinal cancers, actually raised the risk of death. Another study shows vitamin E raises the risk of prostate cancer.

Experts believe it's because antioxidants don't attack cancer cells in the mitochondria part of the cell. That's where cells produce agents that promote tumors. Instead, antioxidants interact with other parts of the cell that don't promote tumors.

Vitamins are "natural" so your doctor doesn't need to know what you take. If you think your vitamin is all-natural, think again. Manufacturers often produce supplements with synthetic additives, then slap the Department of Agriculture's organic seal on the bottles. And it's all legal.

Plus, the Food and Drug Administration doesn't require supplements to undergo rigorous testing like prescription drugs. So the supplement you think you're getting may be spiked with steroids or other ingredients.

Then there's evidence that your supplement can interfere with health conditions, medications, and test results. For instance, vitamin C can botch the outcome of fecal occult blood tests used to detect bleeding in your digestive tract.

Always talk with your doctor about the supplements you take. Buy products with the GMP Certified mark, which stands for "good manufacturing practices." Or look for the USP Verified mark from the nonprofit organization U.S. Pharmacopeia. The supplements with these labels pass tests for strength, quality, purity, and composition.

You can eat anything you want as long as you take a multivitamin. You can't fill up on sugary sweets and saturated fats and expect a multivitamin to undo the damage. And you can't get the fiber found in fruits, veggies, and whole grains, and disease-fighting phytochemicals from a pill. You also need exercise, good sleep, and activities that reduce stress to maintain good health. A supplement can't deliver any of those.

You can't get too much of a good thing. If 100% of the recommended daily allowance is good, then 1,000% should be better —right? Wrong!

- A study out of the Karolinska Institute in Sweden found that men who took 1,000 milligrams of vitamin C are twice as likely to develop kidney stones than those who don't take supplements. In the U.S., the Dietary Reference Intake only recommends 90 milligrams of vitamin C for men and 75 milligrams for women, way below the popular dose of 1,000 milligrams sold in drugstores and supermarkets.

- Take a high dose of vitamin A and your whole body will suffer the consequences. The National Institutes of Health says just one dose of more than 40,000 international units can cause severe headaches, nausea, vertigo, blurred vision, muscle aches, and lack of coordination. Taken repeatedly and you're bound to damage your liver.

- Even water-soluble vitamins — the ones your body flushes out — can wreak havoc on your body if taken in high doses. Vitamin B6 causes heartburn, nausea, skin irritation, sun sensitivity, and severe nerve damage.

Everyone needs a multivitamin. Experts say don't waste your money. Three studies published in the *Annals of Internal Medicine* show multivitamins offer no health benefits to the average person. If you eat a balanced diet loaded with fruits, vegetables, whole grains, and protein — including dairy — then you're getting all the nutrients you need for a healthy life.

Scientists say the only people who might need a multivitamin are pregnant and nursing moms, people who eat less than 1,200 calories a day or cut out complete food groups like carbs, and those who have trouble digesting or absorbing food. Otherwise, talk with your doctor before starting a vitamin supplement. You probably don't need one. And that's a fact.

Tasty kitchen tips to lock in vitamins

It can be tricky — but not impossible — to get fruits and vegetables from farm to table without losing vitamins and minerals. Here's how to protect all those important nutrients when you buy and cook produce.

Pick farm fresh. Not everyone has a farm stand near home. But if you do, locally grown produce packs a powerful punch. That's because fruits and veggies begin to lose their nutrients once they're picked. The sooner you can get your hands on those tomatoes or strawberries, the better.

Don't cast aside cans. If farm fresh is not an option, consider canned. A study published in the *Journal of the Science of Food and Agriculture* shows canned peaches have more vitamin C, antioxidants, and folate than fresh ones. Researchers believe it's because canned peaches are picked and packed as soon as they're ripe. And canning makes nutrients in peaches burst out of cell walls.

Mix up your cooking methods. When it comes to cooking vegetables, what works to keep one vitamin intact may not work for another. Experts say whatever method works for you — baking, boiling, steaming, grilling, or microwaving — that's the one you should choose. But keep frying to a minimum. It's the worst way to preserve nutrients.

Use the following tips to safeguard nutrients as long as possible.

- Store fruits and vegetables in a cool room or in your refrigerator once ripe.

- Place spinach, broccoli, and salad greens in your refrigerator's high-humidity drawer.

- Keep canned goods in a cool place.

- Keep cooking and reheating times to a minimum, and use as little water as possible.

- Leave the skins on fruits and veggies when cooking. You'll find loads of nutrients in and just under the skin.

Minerals

Mighty minerals heal your body from the inside out

You don't only need vitamins for good health. Minerals are just as important. These elements are found in soil and water. They make their way into your body via the fish, plants, and meats you eat, and the liquids you drink.

Scientists divide minerals into two groups — major and trace. Major minerals include calcium, chloride, phosphorus, potassium, sodium, sulfur, and magnesium. Your body needs all of these to maintain good health. But don't knock trace minerals — iodine, iron, zinc, selenium, fluoride, chromium, copper, boron, molybdenum, and manganese. Just because your body only needs tiny amounts of trace minerals doesn't mean they're not as important as the major ones.

Minerals work much like the pump and radiator in your car's engine. Sodium, chloride, and potassium regulate your body's water. Calcium, phosphorus, and magnesium promote healthy bones. And sulfur stabilizes the proteins your body needs for healthy hair, skin, and nails.

But don't forget your brain — minerals charge up your brain like a car battery charges a car. Take magnesium, for example. It guards against memory loss. An animal study from China suggests magnesium threonate — a specially formulated compound — may even reverse the cognitive decline associated with Alzheimer's. A more recent human study shows magnesium threonate supplements increase thinking and reasoning skills and decrease forgetfulness.

Potassium from sources like bananas and potatoes maintains your blood pressure, which protects the lining of the arteries in your brain.

A study published in *Nutrition Journal* says iron supplements could boost your IQ and your ability to pay attention and concentrate. But bear in mind, too much iron can be toxic. Adults over age 65 generally have plenty of iron stored in their bodies. So don't take an iron supplement without checking with your doctor first.

Here are some more details about the critical roles minerals play in your body, and how much you need to get each day in grams (g), milligrams (mg), or micrograms (mcg).

Major minerals

Calcium. By far the most abundant mineral in your body, calcium makes your bones and teeth strong and hard. Without it, they would be as floppy as your ears.

Calcium doesn't just stay trapped in your skeleton, though. Small amounts of it travel into your blood. There, it's essential for steadying your blood pressure and helping your muscles contract. One rather important muscle — your heart — needs calcium to keep pumping.

Calcium is critical during childhood if you want to have strong bones as an adult. But no matter how old you are, it's never too late to get more of this important mineral. Without enough calcium, you can suffer from bone loss, called osteoporosis.

Good sources of calcium include dairy foods, broccoli, kale, small bony fish, and legumes.

Calcium	DRI women	age 51-70	1,200 mg
		age 71+	1,200 mg
	DRI men	age 51-70	1,000 mg
		age 71+	1,200 mg

Chloride. Your stomach would be useless without this element. Chloride is a main ingredient in your digestive stomach acids. It also helps to assure that all of your body's cells get their fair share of nutrients and that your bodily fluids are properly balanced.

Chloride pairs up with sodium to create table salt and sea salt and is often the main ingredient in salt substitutes. You'll also find it in many vegetables, so search the supermarket for foods like lettuce, celery, seaweed, tomatoes, and olives.

Chloride	DRI women	age 51-70	2 g
		age 71+	1.8 g
	DRI men	age 51-70	2 g
		age 71+	1.8 g

Magnesium. This is the least common major mineral in your body, but that doesn't hold magnesium back. First, it helps keep your bones and teeth healthy, then it makes sure calcium, potassium, vitamin D, and proteins do their jobs. When you flex your muscles, you need magnesium to help them relax again.

Researchers have found this superstar mineral may help prevent diabetes, high blood pressure, cancer — even heart attacks.

Because of processed foods and poor soil, magnesium may be the one life-saving mineral you aren't getting enough of. Green leafy vegetables, legumes, seeds, nuts, and whole grains will provide you with a healthy dose. You'll also find it in some breakfast cereals and other fortified foods.

Magnesium	DRI women	age 51+	320 mg
	DRI men	age 51+	420 mg

Phosphorus. The second-most plentiful mineral in your body works hand in hand with calcium to build and maintain strong bones and teeth. Phosphorus is a crucial ingredient in DNA and cell membranes and helps make healthy new cells all over your body. To top it off, phosphorus helps turn your food into energy.

This important mineral is also critical for kidney function, muscle contractions, a normal heartbeat, and nerve signaling.

You'll mainly find it in protein sources like meat and milk along with processed foods that contain sodium phosphate. If you eat plenty of foods that contain calcium and protein, you'll also get enough phosphorus in your diet.

Phosphorus	DRI women	age 51+	700 mg
	DRI men	age 51+	700 mg

Potassium. Keeping your blood pressure steady, maintaining your heartbeat, balancing water in your cells, and assuring your muscles and nerves work properly are a few of potassium's many important jobs. Like magnesium, this mineral might be essential for heart health.

When you write your grocery list, consider foods high in potassium such as baked potatoes and sweet potatoes with skin, prune juice, tomato paste and puree, canned white beans, acorn squash, wild salmon, yogurt, and of course, bananas.

Potassium	DRI women	age 51+	4.7 g
	DRI men	age 51+	4.7 g

Sodium. This mineral usually gets a bad rap because it's the main element in salt. But your body needs sodium to maintain its balance of fluids. It also helps with nerve and muscle function.

Nowadays, most people try to limit their salt, or sodium, intake for health reasons. Those who are salt-sensitive are especially at risk for heart disease. But it would benefit everyone to lower their daily sodium intake to 2,300 milligrams or less — about a teaspoon of table salt.

Remember that most of your sodium comes from packaged and processed foods, not from your salt shaker. You can check the Nutrition Facts label to find out how much sodium is in prepared foods. Among the worst offenders are breads, cold cuts and cured meats, soups, cheese, and snack foods like popcorn, pretzels, chips, and crackers.

Sodium	DRI women	age 51-70	1,300 mg
		age 71+	1,200 mg
	DRI men	age 51-70	1,300 mg
		age 71+	1,200 mg

Sulfur. After calcium and phosphorus, sulfur is the most abundant mineral in your body. It's especially important in proteins because it gives them shape and durability. Your body's toughest proteins — in your hair, nails, and skin — have the highest amounts. Sulfur also helps form healthy cartilage and ligaments.

Foods high in sulfur include eggs, meats, seafood, nuts, milk, cheddar cheese, peaches, broccoli, onions, and garlic. There is no recommended dietary allowance for sulfur.

Trace minerals

Boron. This important trace mineral is essential for bone growth and wound healing. It helps your body produce and use estrogen, testosterone, and vitamin D, and boosts the absorption of magnesium and calcium. Plus it works as an anti-inflammatory to help relieve arthritis. But the biggest benefit may be its demonstrated ability to fight cancer.

Fill up on this mineral by eating noncitrus fruits, raisins, nuts, legumes, and dark leafy greens. No dietary reference intakes have been set.

Chromium. On the verge of diabetes? You may need some help from chromium. This essential trace mineral helps improve the way your body uses insulin. It may also be involved in carbohydrate, fat, and protein metabolism.

Chromium has been studied for its possible connection to various health conditions such as diabetes and weight loss. It is widely used as a supplement, but government guidelines stress that foods should be your primary source.

You'll find chromium in egg yolk, brewer's yeast, broccoli, apples, bananas, grape and orange juice, meats, whole grains, garlic, and basil.

Chromium	DRI women	age 51+	30 mcg
	DRI men	age 51+	20 mcg

Copper. You need this mighty mineral to stay healthy. Your body uses copper to make red blood cells, produce energy, and fight off free radicals. It helps maintain your nervous and immune systems and is important for brain development.

You can get the recommended amounts of copper by eating a variety of foods, including organ meats, seafood, nuts, seeds, whole grains, mushrooms, avocados, chickpeas, and chocolate.

Copper	DRI women	age 51+	900 mcg
	DRI men	age 51+	900 mcg

Fluoride. This trace mineral occurs naturally in your body as calcium fluoride and is mostly found in your bones and teeth. Fluoride helps reduce tooth decay. Studies have found that adding it to tap water helps cut cavities in children by more than half.

Most communities add fluoride to their water systems, so drinking tap water should give you an adequate amount. The ocean contains natural sodium fluoride so most seafood will have it. You'll also find it in tea and gelatin and in foods prepared or processed with fluoridated water.

Fluoride	DRI women	age 51+	3 mg
	DRI men	age 51+	4 mg

Iodine. Your body needs iodine to make thyroid hormones. These hormones control your metabolism and many other important functions. They also contribute to proper bone and brain development during pregnancy and infancy.

Buying iodized salt is a good way to make sure you get enough iodine in your diet. You can also get it naturally through seafood, seaweed, dairy products, breads, and cereals.

Iodine	DRI women	age 51+	150 mcg
	DRI men	age 51+	150 mcg

Iron. Without a teaspoon of this mineral in your body, you couldn't breathe. Iron makes up hemoglobin and myoglobin, two compounds that carry oxygen throughout your blood and your muscles. No wonder you feel weak and listless when you are iron deficient.

Iron is critical for red blood cell formation, growth and development, immune function, reproduction, and wound healing. You'll find it in meats, poultry, seafood, beans and peas, dark green vegetables, prunes, and fortified cereals and breads.

Iron	DRI women	age 51+	8 mg
	DRI men	age 51+	8 mg

Manganese. This important trace mineral helps you process carbohydrates, protein, and cholesterol as well as form cartilage and bone. It also plays a role in blood clotting to promote wound healing.

Manganese shows up in a wide variety of foods, including whole grains, nuts, soybeans and other legumes, leafy vegetables, oysters, clams, mussels, rice, coffee, tea, and many spices, such as black pepper.

Manganese	DRI women	age 51+	1.8 mg
	DRI men	age 51+	2.3 mg

Molybdenum. You need this small but mighty mineral for optimal health. Your body uses molybdenum to process proteins and genetic material like DNA. It also helps break down drugs and toxic substances that enter your body.

The amount of molybdenum in food depends on how much is in the soil. Your best bet is to eat a variety of foods like legumes, whole grains, rice, nuts, potatoes, bananas, leafy vegetables, milk, yogurt, cheese, beef, chicken, and eggs.

Molybdenum	DRI women	age 51+	45 mcg
	DRI men	age 51+	45 mcg

Selenium. This trace mineral carries out important daily tasks in your body. It helps your thyroid use iodine, for instance, and it's important for a healthy immune system. A deficiency in selenium can cause heart and thyroid disease.

Selenium is found naturally in plants and animal products, but the amount depends on how much was in the soil the plants were grown in and the foods the animals ate. Eat plenty of whole grains, seeds, nuts — especially Brazil nuts — meat, poultry, eggs, and seafood to make sure you're getting enough.

Selenium	DRI women	age 51+	55 mcg
	DRI men	age 51+	55 mcg

Zinc. Want to stay healthy? Make sure you get enough zinc in your diet. Cleaning up free radicals, building new cells, and creating energy are just three of the jobs zinc has in your body.

This mineral also helps your immune system fight off invading bacteria and viruses that cause infections. It heals wounds and sharpens your sense of taste and smell. Plus research suggests zinc might help fight macular degeneration.

If you love shellfish, eat up. Oysters, clams, crabs, and lobsters are good sources of zinc. You'll also find it in beef, poultry, fortified cereals, beans, and nuts.

Zinc	DRI women	age 51+	8 mg
	DRI men	age 51+	11 mg

Phytochemicals

Powerful plant chemicals wage war on disease

Natural compounds in plants, called phytochemicals or phytonutrients, can have an amazing effect on your body. These tens of thousands of substances — found in fruits, vegetables, herbs, and spices — are not considered essential nutrients like vitamins, minerals, fat, protein, and carbohydrates, but they still play an important role in your health.

Unlock nature's amazing defenses. Some specific phytochemicals do more than one kind of job. Here are just a few of the many benefits.

- block cancer-causing substances in the food you eat and air you breathe

- lower the inflammation that triggers cancer cell growth

- curb the growth rate of cancer cells

- help your body regulate hormones

- lower blood pressure

- fight bad bacteria

- reduce cholesterol

- battle brain disorders

- protect your vision

- reduce stroke risk

> No Dietary Reference Intakes (DRIs) exist for phytochemicals. Experts simply recommend you eat a diet rich in fruits and vegetables to get enough of these important compounds.

Enjoy a rainbow of fruits and vegetables. Part of their purpose is to protect plants from weather, pests, and other dangers. But phytochemicals are also responsible for certain scents, colors, and flavors. That's why you'll find brightly colored produce are often the richest sources of these beneficial plant chemicals.

There are so many phytochemicals, scientists have broken them into classes, based on chemical structure, and then subgroups. For instance, carotenoids are a group of over 600 dyes found in plants that provide color ranging from light yellow to red. Flavonoids are another group of more than 4,000 plant pigments that give many flowers and herbs their yellow, orange, and red color. And anthocyanins give foods their blue, red, or purple colors.

Whole foods are your wisest choice. Many cultures, like the Chinese and American Indians, have always looked to plants for healing. Even today, the World Health Organization says about 80% of the people on earth use natural medicine — mostly involving plants.

However, modern man's passion for science and advanced technology has inflated the market for pills and capsules, replacing whole sources of nutrition. That's why you'll find a host of supplements in stores and on the internet offering an easy supply of phytochemicals.

But there is very little evidence these plant chemicals do the same job once you take them out of their original "package," possibly because the chemicals need other parts of the plant to work properly. As always, the best way for you to get the most benefit from phytochemicals is to eat whole foods.

To make the most of these natural medicines, choose lots of fruit, double the amount of vegetables you normally eat, season your dishes with herbs and spices, and plan several meatless meals that contain legumes and whole grains. In addition, cook your vegetables lightly since heat destroys many of these healthful substances.

Type	Food sources	Possible benefits
Anthocyanins (such as cyanidin, delphinidin)	• chickpeas • blackberries • currants • strawberries • black grapes	fights heart disease, cancer, and diabetes; improves eye health; helps control weight gain; shows antibacterial and antimicrobial activity
Carotenoids (such as beta carotene, lycopene, lutein, zeaxanthin)	• broccoli • carrots • cooked tomatoes • leafy greens • sweet potatoes • winter squash • apricots • cantaloupe • oranges • watermelon	works as an antioxidant, fights age-related macular degeneration and cataracts, improves cognitive function, boosts heart health, possibly helps prevent some types of cancer
Flavanols (such as catechin, epicatechin, epigallocatechin, proanthocyani-dins)	• green tea • black tea • dark chocolate • blackberries • cocoa powder • pecans	combats cancer, lowers blood pressure, fights weight gain, reverses memory loss
Flavonols (such as quercetin, kaempferol, myricetin)	• apples • cranberries • radish • red onions • cooked asparagus	provides antioxidant protection against cell damage, lowers blood pressure, protects against inflammation
Indoles and glucosinolates (such as sulforaphane)	• broccoli • cabbage • collard greens • kale • cauliflower • Brussels sprouts	limits production of cancer-related hormones, blocks carcinogens, prevents tumor growth

Type	Food sources	Possible benefits
Inositol (such as phytic acid)	• bran from corn, oats, rice, rye, and wheat • nuts • soybeans and soy products like tofu, soy milk, and edamame	slows cell growth, works as an antioxidant
Isoflavones (such as daidzein, genistein)	• soybeans and soy products like tofu, soy milk, and edamame	protects against cancer, particularly breast and prostate cancer; limits production of cancer-related hormones; may increase bone density; generally works as an antioxidant
Isothiocyanates	• broccoli • cabbage • collard greens • kale • cauliflower • Brussels sprouts	detoxifies cancer-related agents, blocks tumor growth, works as an antioxidant
Polyphenols (such as ellagic acid, resveratrol)	• green tea • grapes and wine • berries • citrus fruits • apples • whole grains • peanuts	prevents cancer formation, prevents inflammation, works as an antioxidant

Big benefits from 5 little-known nutrients

Many phytochemicals make headlines. Others you never hear about, but they're just as important for your health. Here's a look at a few of them and their powerful perks.

Limonene. This tangy nutrient clobbers cancer cells and keeps them from spreading. You find these in lime, lemon, orange, grapefruit, and tangerine peels. But if eating peels doesn't sound, well, appealing, you can toss lemon zest into pasta, make candied peels, or create your own citrus salt.

Sterols and stanols. They look like cholesterol but do more good than harm. Plant sterols block bad fats from getting absorbed by your intestines. The results? Lower LDL cholesterol. Add them to your diet by switching over to sterol-fortified spreads or orange juice. Or eat asparagus, nuts and seeds, and whole grains.

Tannins. What do tea, cider, and chickpeas have in common? They all tackle cancer cells and stop them from wreaking havoc with your health. That's because they contain tannins — cancer-fighters with antioxidant abilities.

Organosulfur. If you love the pungent flavors of chives, onions, and garlic, you're in luck. These flavorful foods trigger your body's defenses against cancer. And here's a tip for garlic-lovers. Chopping or crushing garlic 10 minutes before cooking it boosts its cancer-fighting compounds.

Chlorogenic acid. Java lovers take note. Coffee is loaded with chlorogenic acid — a phytochemical that protects your central nervous system from degenerative nerve diseases like Alzheimer's and Parkinson's. And you don't have to drink caffeinated joe for this health perk. Decaf serves up the same protection.

Probiotics

Bugs with benefits: Good health begins with probiotics

Bacteria have gotten a bad rap. You probably think of them as germs. And, in many cases, you would be right. But bacteria that live and thrive inside your body are so much more.

Your digestive system, especially, is home to an abundance of bacteria that help it work properly. These are sometimes called gut flora or intestinal microbiota. They help you digest, absorb, synthesize, and metabolize all kinds of nutrients and other substances. When you don't have enough good bacteria here you can often feel it, in the form of constipation, gas, diarrhea, or various infections.

But scientists are continuing to explore other areas of the body containing good bacteria and just how these microorganisms — known collectively as your microbiome — impact your health, including some of these common conditions.

> Your digestive tract contains 100 trillion bacterial cells. These make up your intestinal microbiome and are vital to your overall health.

- sinusitis
- high cholesterol
- rheumatoid arthritis
- memory loss
- allergies
- high blood pressure
- obesity

You can buy probiotics, which are live microorganisms similar to the ones you have naturally in your body. They come as capsules, tablets, or powders, and in certain foods, like yogurt. You would want to take probiotics for several reasons.

- to generally boost your immune system

- to replace the good bacteria killed off by disease, stress, poor diet, or a round of antibiotics

- to treat or prevent certain conditions or infections

When choosing a probiotic, select one with the type of bacteria shown to work for your complaint. Next, make sure you're getting enough live cells in every dose. Products can range from 100 million cells to 900 billion per dose. You'll have to do your homework here to determine what you need. And finally, remember there are some situations where taking probiotics is not a healthy decision, so talk to your doctor first.

Surprising way to boost friendly gut flora

Probiotics need something to eat, and they love to feast on certain types of fiber. Experts call this fiber a "prebiotic" since it isn't fully digested and can hang around in your intestines, feeding your probiotics. That keeps you and your gut healthy.

While not all prebiotics are carbohydrates, the major ones are from a group called oligosaccharide carbohydrates (OSCs), and are found naturally in tasty foods like these.

asparagus	bananas	barley
beans	chicory	cow's milk
garlic	honey	Jerusalem artichokes
onions	peas	rye
seaweeds	soybean	sugar beets
tomatoes	wheat	

When the good bacteria in your intestines feed on these prebiotics, they break them down into very small molecules called short-chain fatty acids (SCFAs). These enter your bloodstream and travel throughout your body, influencing not only your gastrointestinal system but protecting you from a whole host of disorders. Among other benefits, they also have these powerful effects.

- boost your immune system
- lower inflammation
- promote healthy blood sugar levels by improving insulin resistance
- fight bad bacteria

And by encouraging the growth of probiotics, they help your body control obesity, irritable bowel syndrome, inflammatory bowel disease, depression, and heart disease.

The International Scientific Association for Probiotics and Prebiotics suggests you get at least 5 grams of prebiotics every day. While you can get some from food, you may want to take supplements or eat products with added prebiotics, like certain yogurts, cereals, bread, or drinks.

You won't always see the word "prebiotic" on the label so look for these terms.

- galactooligosaccharides (GOS)
- fructooligosaccharides (FOS)
- oligofructose (OF)
- chicory fiber
- inulin

Water

Tap into the simple healing power of water

Water is more essential to life than any other single nutrient on this planet. You could live without food for a month or more, but you can only live a couple of days without water.

It has no calories, no fat, and no sugar. It doesn't need processing by your digestive system, and it's helpful to most of your body's functions.

For instance, it's the "juice" that keeps your chemical processes going. It dissolves minerals, vitamins, and other nutrients and carries them to where you need them. And it helps form the structure of your cells, tissues, and organs.

It's everywhere, part of every living thing, and the world's most perfect beverage.

Beware the dangers of dehydration. When the percentage of water in your body begins to fall below normal, you start becoming dehydrated. It's a vague condition to most people — you may think it is simply feeling thirsty. However, by the time you actually feel thirsty, you're already in need of water and will soon start feeling the effects. These can range from simply annoying to dangerous.

- headache
- lack of concentration
- dry lips and mouth
- rapid breathing
- dark urine
- seizures
- death

- fatigue
- dizziness
- a faster heart rate
- confusion
- shock
- coma

Hard to believe you could get into that much trouble simply by not drinking enough water, but dehydration can be a sneaky condition, creeping up without much warning. This is especially true for older people.

First of all, certain drugs can dehydrate you before you know it. But also as you age, you lose some of your feelings of thirst, and so might not notice that you need a drink. In addition, your kidneys are older and not as efficient at keeping water in your body.

Stay sharp and energized. Even though losing 5% of your water weight is a standard benchmark for dehydration, losing just 2% of your body's water weight can affect the way you feel, think, and act. Someone weighing 200 pounds would notice a difference if they lost even 2 1/2 pounds of water.

The Institute of Medicine once recommended about 11 cups of fluids for women and almost 16 cups for men. But the right amount also depends on things like how much you sweat and how much water you get from foods like soup, juice, herbal tea, nonfat milk, fruits, and vegetables. That's why experts no longer strictly endorse eight glasses of water daily.

Tests showed that people suffering this degree of dehydration scored lower on math skills, lost short-term memory abilities, were slower to make decisions, and were generally more fatigued than people with plenty of water to drink.

In another recent study, mildly dehydrated young women were less able to concentrate, found tasks more difficult, felt more fatigued and angry, and were more prone to headaches. When young men were mildly dehydrated, they became less vigilant, had poorer working memory, and felt more tired and anxious.

Slim down with the great soda swap

Want to cut calories and save money? Drink more water —
especially instead of diet-busting sugary sodas, which average
about 160 calories or 10 teaspoons of sugar a can.

Experts know sipping H2O is an easy but important way to
curb your appetite. Drink up about an hour before you eat,
and drink lots with every meal. You will feel more full and eat
more slowly because of it. The best news — water is a natural,
safer alternative to diet pills.

And amazingly, a gallon of drinking water from your kitchen
faucet costs less than a penny, according to the American
Water Works Association. That's right. Less than 1 cent. The
average American family spends an estimated $850 every
year on those calorie-laden soft drinks. You do the math.

Wash away your top health hazards

Water, that wonderfully healthy, natural refreshment, is now the
most popular beverage in the United States. Find out why it's just
what you need to feel better and stay well.

- Your heart pumps blood through your body more easily
  when you drink enough water. One study even suggests five
  glasses a day may lower your risk of a heart attack.

- Treat yourself with water to help eliminate your arthritis
  pain. Without enough water, increased friction between
  joints can mean more swelling, stiffness, and pain. Drink
  water to lubricate and cushion your joints and transport the
  nutrients they need.

- The buildup of uric acid causes gout, another kind of arthritis. Studies show drinking water flushes out uric acid and helps prevent painful gout attacks.

- If your digestive system is plagued with problems, make water your No. 1 priority. Whether it is constipation, heartburn, irritable bowel syndrome, or just plain indigestion, lots of water will soothe your system and get things moving in the right direction.

- Water dissolves the calcium in your urine that can turn into kidney stones. Plus it helps the bile in your liver dissolve cholesterol that could become painful gallstones.

- Drinking at least 17 ounces of water a day — just over 2 cups — may cut your risk of high blood sugar and diabetes.

- Water helps prevent cavities by washing away acid-producing food.

- Fight bladder cancer by flushing out cancer-causing substances.

Pinch and press — 2 ways to test hydration

Not sure if you're dried up? Try one of these tests to see if it's time to break out the water bottle.

Skin pinch. Dehydration can curb your skin's ability to change shape and return to normal, known as skin elasticity. Gently pinch some skin on the back of your hand and stretch it up. When you release, the skin should bounce back into position.

Nail press. This test monitors blood flow to your tissues, which is a marker of hydration. Hold your hand above your heart. Apply pressure to your nail bed until it turns white, indicating that the blood has left the tissue. Remove pressure. If it takes longer than two seconds for the pink color to return, you may be dehydrated.

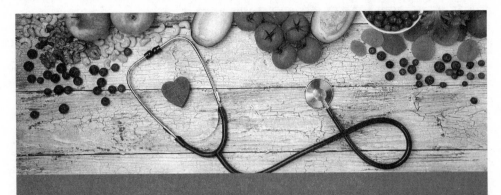

Eat to beat disease:
Kitchen cures that help your body heal

Open your pantry and take a peek. What do you see?
Cartons of empty calories that will only temporarily satisfy
your cravings, or containers of life-giving nutrients
guaranteed to bolster your body?

Healthy eating habits go hand in hand with a healthy life.
What you put in your body can encourage or combat life-
threatening diseases. Discover the very best veggies, fruits,
spices, and oils to fend off heart disease, boost your
brainpower, soothe your joints, and more. Yes, food can
do that.

Age-related macular degeneration

Double up on protection with this dynamic duo

Great things come in pairs. Just think of salt and pepper, peanut butter and jelly, and lutein and zeaxanthin. OK, so that last one may not be as famous, but if you're looking for eye protection, it's hard to top this dynamic duo.

Lutein and zeaxanthin are naturally occurring plant chemicals. They help protect your orbs from light-induced damage that can break down your macula, the central part of the retina with your sharpest vision. That can result in age-related macular degeneration (AMD), a leading cause of blindness.

AMD usually begins in the late 50s or 60s and is likely to occur in one-third of people over age 75. High risk factors are smoking, light-colored eyes, longtime sun exposure, high blood pressure, heart disease, and family history of AMD or heart disease.

Large studies revealed that eating foods rich in lutein and zeaxanthin can help slash your risk of developing this irreversible disease. So how can you get more of this powerful pair in your diet?

Try an exotic fruit to slash your risk of AMD. Goji berries, sometimes also called wolfberries, hail from the far east. This exotic fruit is prized for more than its sweet-and-sour taste. It's chock-full of lutein and zeaxanthin as well as other powerful antioxidants. And experts think goji berries are a great way to ward off AMD.

Eat

Avocado	Goji berries
Collard greens	Beets
Fatty fish	Cantaloupe
Olive oil	Oranges
Kiwis	Almond milk
Fortified cereal	Eggs

Avoid

Foods high in fat, like french fries and hamburgers

In a recent study, researchers divided 114 seniors with early AMD into two groups. Half of them added 25 grams, or about 5 tablespoons, of goji berries to their diet for 90 days while the others stuck with their normal diet. At the end of the study, those who ate goji berries had better vision and higher levels of zeaxanthin in their eyes.

Look for dried goji berries at your local supermarket. If they're not in stock, tangerines and dried peaches are another great source of these sight-saving nutrients.

Don't miss this soul food staple that could save your aging vision. Over 60? You might want to take a sojourn to the south to seek out one of the best foods for your eyes — collard greens.

These dark leafy greens are packed with lutein and zeaxanthin. And studies show that people who eat more of these nutrients are less likely to get AMD. Experts suggest eating around 12 milligrams (mg) of these nutrients combined every day. You'll get more than that in a cup of cooked collards.

Not a fan of collard greens? Don't fret. Most dark, leafy green veggies will do. Spinach and kale are both excellent sources of these powerful antioxidants.

> Can't seem to get enough lutein through diet alone? You might want to consider a supplement. However, they're not all created equal. Look for lutein that's labeled as "free form." Your body is better at absorbing and using that specific form of the antioxidant.

'Beet' AMD by adding a single food to your diet

Could a single vegetable like beetroot hold the secret to slashing your risk of age-related macular degeneration? Experts think it could help.

Scientists asked more than 3,500 people about the foods they ate most often. And over the course of 15 years, the researchers regularly examined participants' eyes for signs of vision loss.

The study revealed that the people who ate 100 to 142 milligrams (mg) of vegetable nitrates each day were 35% less likely to develop early AMD compared to those who ate the least. Eating more nitrates did not make a significant difference.

Nitrates are important because they turn into nitric oxide, which plays a critical role in maintaining good blood flow throughout your body, including your eyes. They also help fight off the oxidative damage that causes your vision to fade over the years.

Beets are one of the top sources of nitrates. They have nearly 15 mg of nitrates per 100 grams, so a can of beets will get you two-thirds of the way there. Eat them cold in a salad with other nitrate-rich veggies like spinach, cabbage, and radishes, or heat them up for a tangy side dish. Your eyes will thank you.

The 'eyes' have it — vote for healthy fats to save your sight

You probably know that sitting down to a dinner of french fries, hamburgers, and milkshakes isn't great for your heart. But did you know a high-fat diet could harm your vision, too?

All those bad fats alter your gut bacteria, which causes inflammation throughout your body. In turn, your eyes are more at risk for damage that eventually causes age-related macular degeneration (AMD).

But that doesn't mean all fat is bad. In fact, the right fats can help you protect your eyes. So swap those unhealthy foods for these tasty treats.

Cut your risk of eye disease nearly in half with fishy delights.
They say you are what you eat, and your eyes are no exception. The retina, the light-sensitive layer at the back of your eyeball,

is chock-full of omega-3 fatty acids. And studies have found that eating omega-3 foods is linked to a lower risk of cataracts and AMD. How?

- Omega-3 clobbers inflammation that can harm your retinas, contributing to AMD.

- These nutrients also pump up your good cholesterol, which ferries powerful antioxidants — like vitamin E — to your eyes, where they fight off damage associated with cataracts.

You can keep your vision sharp into your 90s by snacking on the right foods. In fact, one study shows that eating two or more servings of fatty fish each week — like salmon, sardines, and albacore tuna — can slash your risk of AMD by almost 50%.

Keep your eyesight sharper than Superman with this super snack. Avocados contain lutein and zeaxanthin, which means they can help protect your eyes from harmful blue light. And experts say this tasty, delicious treat is one of the best ways to protect your eyesight. Bring on the guacamole.

But the real secret may not be the nutrients in this fantastic fruit. An avocado actually contains less lutein and zeaxanthin than leafy greens like spinach. But a recent study revealed it's a superstar at increasing the amount of antioxidants in your eyes. The reason? Avocado's healthy fats help your body absorb and use all those nutrients.

Protect your eyes with a virtual trip to the Mediterranean. French researchers examined the diets and eye health of over 650 seniors. They found that those who regularly used olive oil were significantly less likely to develop late AMD, an advanced form of the disease.

The reason? Olive oil is loaded with a chemical called oleocanthal. This compound works like over-the-counter painkillers to fight off inflammation. A steady dose of this natural anti-inflammatory over time may help protect your eyes from the damage that causes AMD.

Researchers also noted that most seniors likely used extra-virgin olive oil, which is higher in protective antioxidants than regular olive oil. Perfect for salad dressings or sauteing your delicious Mediterranean veggies.

Give grandma's collards a healthier twist

Collard greens are a staple on every southern table. Traditionally, this hardy vegetable is simmered for hours until nice and tender. But there's one problem with that — most of the nutrients either leach into the cooking liquid or are destroyed by the heat.

Sure, you can sop up the cooking liquid with cornbread. But a better idea is to bring grandma's recipe into the 21st century by quick-steaming the collards with a pressure cooker. That's the perfect way to preserve all those wonderful nutrients.

Just put water and a steaming basket in your pressure cooker, add the greens, and set your timer to zero. It will shut off as soon as it reaches cooking pressure. Twist the valve to release the steam. That's it. You'll have perfectly cooked greens that are still chock-full of vitamins, minerals, and antioxidants.

Don't have a pressure cooker? Simply steam your greens in a pot on the stove.

Want to keep your vision sharp? Fill up with these fruits

You're familiar with the old saying, "an apple a day keeps the doctor away." But what if you want to keep the eye doctor at bay? New research says apples might not be your best bet. Instead, consider calling on a few other powerful fruits.

Protect yourself from the top two sight-stealers with a sweet, delicious melon. You may have heard that eating carrots can help you see better at night. Believe it or not, that was a myth created by the British air force during WWII to hide the fact they could pick out German bombers at night with radar.

So what's the truth? Orange foods — like cantaloupe, sweet potatoes, and carrots — are high in beta carotene, a vital nutrient for healthy eyes. A recent study conducted by New Zealand-based researchers discovered that a diet rich in beta carotene may help ward off AMD and cataracts. Experts say beta carotene acts as a powerful antioxidant, meaning it neutralizes this damage to keep your eyes healthy.

Women should aim for 700 micrograms (mcg) of beta carotene a day, and men, 900 mcg. You can get all the sight-saving nutrients you need in 1 cup of cantaloupe. Eat it regularly to slash your risk of macular degeneration and cataracts.

Two more fruits that should top your list. You might load up on vitamin C when you're trying to ward off a cold or the flu. Here's another reason to pump up the C. It might be just what you need to keep your peepers in tiptop shape.

According to a study published in the *American Journal of Clinical Nutrition*, simply eating a single orange a day can reduce your risk of AMD by almost 60% compared to eating no oranges at all. That's because its vitamin C — a potent antioxidant — helps ward off the oxidative stress that damages your eyes and saps you of your sight.

If you want to add something different to your diet, consider the succulent kiwi. Some kiwifruits have as much vitamin C as two oranges, the potassium strength of a banana, and as much fiber as many whole-grain cereals. Look for Zespri sungolds in addition to the usual green variety.

Brew up some powerful protection for your peepers

One of the best things to do on a rainy day is sit down with a good book and a piping hot cup of tea. But if AMD is robbing you of your sight, reading might not be as fun as it used to be. Symptoms include a gradual blurring or blind spot in your central field of vision, making it hard to read printed words.

Fortunately, you can keep your eyesight keen as you age with a fragrant tea that's loaded with vision-protecting nutrients. Surprise, it's not green or black — it's red.

Rooibos tea — made from the roots of the South African shrub *aspalathus linearis* — is packed with antioxidants. Researchers think this exotic tea is particularly effective at fighting off oxidative damage in your eyes, which means it's perfect protection against AMD.

You can pick up this super tea at most grocery stores. If you can't find it, look for it online.

Open your eyes to a better breakfast

Want to start your day off right? A big bowl of fortified cereal topped with almond milk is the way to go, especially if you're trying to ward off vision loss. Here's why.

Help out your headlights with this mighty mineral. A large trial, known as the Age-Related Eye Disease Study (AREDS), found a combo of nutrients that could lower your odds of developing advanced AMD. Zinc was one of the powerful ingredients singled out by researchers.

But it doesn't work alone. That's why the American Optometric Association calls it the "helper molecule." It ferries vitamin A to your eyes where it helps create the pigments that protect your peepers.

Experts recommend about 11 milligrams (mg) of zinc each day. A single serving of fortified cereal will get you there. And you can get even more in foods like beef, crab, or oysters.

Get some "E"xcellent protection for your eyes with this super vitamin. Researchers also singled out vitamin E in the AREDS trials. That's because this powerful antioxidant helps quash your risk of developing AMD. How? It protects cells from the damage free radicals cause that leads to vision loss.

Almond milk is loaded with this nutrient, and a cup will get you about halfway to your daily requirement of 15 mg. Even better? Some cereals are fortified with vitamin E, so you can get a double dose with breakfast.

Bone up on calcium for stronger peepers. A recent study in *JAMA Ophthalmology* analyzed AREDS participants, and this is what researchers found.

- Those who ate the most calcium-rich foods also had the lowest risk of developing late AMD, compared to people who ate the least.

- And taking calcium supplements seemed to help fight off the wet form of AMD, where abnormal blood vessels grow and leak under the macula, destroying your central vision.

The researchers were not sure exactly how calcium protects your eyes and emphasized that the link needs further study. But it doesn't hurt to make sure you get enough each day. That means at least 1,200 mg for women and 1,000 mg for men.

The cup of almond milk you put in your cereal will get you about 20% of your daily requirement. Other good sources include yogurt, cheese, leafy greens, and even fortified orange juice.

Fend off AMD with this sight-saving supplement

The landmark Age-Related Eye Disease Study (AREDS) found that a supplement of vitamin E, beta carotene, vitamin C, and zinc could slow the progression of AMD by up to 25%.

Unfortunately, beta carotene supplements increase the risk of cancer in smokers. So a new formula — dubbed AREDS 2 — swaps it out for lutein and zeaxanthin. And the research shows this combination is just as powerful. Simply look for AREDS 2 supplements at your local grocery store or online.

Talk to your doctor first if you're considering taking this multivitamin. You could find that you already get most — if not all — of these nutrients in your diet.

Fight eye disease with a little pot of gold

Good eyesight makes you appreciate the beautiful colors of a rainbow, and it may even help you find the proverbial pot of gold. But your eyes will be richer if you look for golden foods instead — and orange, red, and green ones, too.

Surprisingly, the little golden egg yolk is one of the best sources of the carotenoids lutein and zeaxanthin. And because of the yolk's fat content, your body absorbs these eye-saving nutrients more easily than from other sources.

Researchers suggest that if you've given up eggs in the past, you might want to reconsider. To be on the safe side, if you eat more eggs, cut out an equal amount of saturated fat somewhere else in your diet. Try eating less meat or whole dairy products.

Allergies

Snack your way through hay fever season with a tangy treat

You've kept all of your windows closed and worn a mask outside, but you're still reaching for a tissue to catch your runny nose. Outsmart your allergies a different way by reaching for a creamy probiotic snack that's probably already in your fridge.

Balance your allergy response with good bugs. When you come in contact with an allergen — pollen or dust, for example — your immune system overreacts by making antibodies. These antibodies trigger the release of histamines and other chemicals that cause inflammation. Next thing you know, your nose is stuffy, your eyes itch and water, and you start sneezing.

Researchers think the less variety of bacteria you have in your gut, the higher your risk of developing those irritating symptoms. So it's probiotics to the rescue. These beneficial bacteria boost the number of regulatory T-cells in your body, which helps balance your immune system. And — voila — you may not feel quite so lousy anymore.

Spoon up season-long benefits with yogurt. Participants in a recent eight week study conducted during spring allergy season reported better quality of life, including fewer allergy symptoms, after taking probiotic supplements. The supplements contained *Lactobacillus gasseri*, *Bifidobacterium bifidum*, and *Bifidobacterium longum*, but additional studies have found success with other strains of probiotics so researchers are still working on identifying the best types to aid your allergies.

Eat
Yogurt
Probiotic drinks
Nutritional yeast

Avoid
Foods that trigger pollen allergies, which might include nuts and celery

In the meantime, you can find a range of live probiotics packed into yogurt. Before you buy, check the label for the "best by" date because live cultures die off over time. Also look for the words "contains" — not "made with" — "live and active cultures," which assures you the beneficial cultures weren't destroyed during processing.

Need allergy relief? Nutritional yeast rises to the challenge

Fashionable "hayfeverites" in 19th century America, unlucky enough have ragweed allergies, used their malady to escape to hay fever resorts. There, they enjoyed a holiday away from the pesky summer pollen. Unfortunately, that's not an option for many suffering the pangs of postnasal drip today. Not to worry — modern hayfeverites can seek affordable relief in their kitchens.

Dietary yeast, created from a species of yeast called *Saccharomyces cerevisiae*, comes in three forms.

- Nutritional yeast is a dried and deactivated form sold as flakes or powder. You can add it directly to your food.

- Brewer's yeast, also deactivated, is bitter to the taste and often comes in supplement form.

- Baker's yeast is granulated and active, which is what makes your bread rise.

Dietary yeast contains beta glucans, soluble fibers that naturally boost your immune system by delivering an anti-inflammatory and antimicrobial double punch.

In one small study, people with ragweed allergies took a daily beta glucan supplement extracted from a strain of baker's yeast. The result after four weeks — fewer runny noses and itchy eyes. Experts say you can get the same amount of beta glucans used in the study from something far yummier for only about five cents a day — a teaspoon of nutritional yeast.

Nutritional yeast is generally safe for most people, but it could aggravate symptoms if you have Crohn's disease or migraines.

Sub nutritional yeast into your favorite cheesy dishes

Are your allergies making you cry? Shake them off with a little nooch — nutritional yeast that adds a delicious cheesy flavor, as well as nutrients, to your plate.

Also known as yeshi, brufax, or savory yeast, you'll just call it a treat for your taste buds when you sprinkle it over your spaghetti.

Look for nutritional yeast in the bulk bin at your grocery store, bottled in the spice aisle, or packaged online.

Next, let your imagination soar. When you need a hint of nuts or a dollop of cheese, try substituting nutritional yeast.

- Blend it with beans in a layered vegetable salad.

- Whip it up in a cheese sauce for pasta.

- Sample it in vegan queso over nachos.

- Add it to soup before serving.

- Sneak it in for a healthy mac and cheese.

- Cook it into twice-baked potatoes.

- Sprinkle it on popcorn.

Opt out of a raw deal: Cook foods to calm this pollen-related reaction

Can you enjoy peach preserves no problem but your mouth tingles after eating a raw peach? More than half of people with hay fever have a similar experience, called oral allergy syndrome.

The reaction happens when your body confuses the proteins in fruits and vegetables with similar proteins found in pollen. Even eating foods that aren't generally linked to allergies can cause itching and swelling in your mouth or throat.

But if you properly prepare trigger foods, you may not have to choose between an uncomfortable reaction and losing out on important nutrients from produce staples like tomatoes, carrots, zucchini, apples, and pears.

That's because cooking or processing changes the protein structure so your body won't recognize it as similar to pollen. Simply try steaming, boiling, canning, broiling, microwaving, or baking your fruits and veggies.

Celery, walnuts, and peanuts stubbornly resist this intervention, so avoid them if they cause symptoms.

Asthma

Why a plant-based diet is nothing to wheeze at

Experts say the key to fending off an asthma attack is treating a flare-up early. But what if you could stop one before it began by simply changing your food choices?

Saturated fat, sodium, and sugar — standard in the American diet — can lower your asthma control. On the other hand, a plant-based diet rich in nutrients helps you build up your internal defenses to resist asthma triggers in the first place.

Amp up on antioxidants to breathe easy. People with asthma often have lower levels of antioxidants in their blood than healthy people. But researchers suggest that eating more than five servings of vegetables and two servings of fruits — the best sources of these antioxidants — each day can give you more control of your asthma.

Working more nutrients into your diet is as simple as opting for steamed collard greens topped with slivered almonds instead of iceberg lettuce. Trade the fries for a sweet potato. Slice up a tomato and steam a squash to complete a meal loaded with the carotenoids, vitamin C, and vitamin E that can set you on a course to breathe easier.

Still not sure? A recent study of 969 adults over an average seven-year period revealed that a high-quality diet — including vegetables, fruits, nuts, and legumes — was associated with less wheezing, chest tightness, and shortness of breath.

Eat
Broccoli
Water
Tomatoes
Sweet potatoes
Salmon
Almonds
Squash

Avoid
Cured and processed meats, such as ham, bacon, and sausage

High-sodium foods

Soda and other drinks with high fructose corn syrup

Feast on fiber to reinforce your airways. Adding extra plant food to your plate also increases your fiber. That's great news for your lungs, say researchers in France.

They analyzed more than 35,000 participants and discovered that those who got plenty of soluble and insoluble fiber had fewer asthma symptoms. Folks who ate more fiber from cereal, fruit, and seeds fared the best.

When your gut bacteria ferment fiber, they produce inflammation fighters called short-chain fatty acids. But these fatty acids don't just stay in your gut. Your body uses them to fight inflammation all over your body — including your lungs, where inflammation makes your airways more sensitive to asthma triggers.

The bottom line? Keep your inhaler nearby, but maybe you won't need to use it so much once you're filling up on antioxidant-packed, fiber-filled fruits and vegetables.

Pollution solution: Soothe your airways with broccoli

It's 5 p.m. somewhere — time for the daily commute. Are you more concerned about traffic congestion or what air pollution might be doing to your airways? If you have asthma, pollution that seeps in through your car's ventilation system can trigger inflammation and worsen symptoms.

Fortunately, you can arm yourself against rush-hour pollutants by eating broccoli throughout the week. According to one study, the sulforaphane provided in about a cup of cooked broccoli can boost your cells' antioxidant ability and your anti-inflammatory response to air pollutants.

Broccoli also has quercetin, which puts the brakes on your body's histamine production and blocks inflammation.

Stop bringing home the bacon and breathe easier

Country-fried ham, bacon, and sausage might sound like the start of an amazing Saturday morning breakfast, but they could also be an invitation to an asthma attack.

Researchers found in a study of over 35,000 people that eating processed meat was associated with more asthma symptoms, especially when participants were overweight, eating a lower quality diet, or smoking.

Why? For one, when you eat cured meats, the amount of C-reactive proteins in your body goes up, which means more inflammation and possibly more trouble breathing. To make things worse, cured meats are packed with three ingredients that aggravate asthma.

- **Nitrites.** These are preservatives that prolong the shelf life of your meat. While nitrites alone are not the bad guys, they can turn on you in a flash when cooked in high heat. That's when they convert to nitrosamines, which may cause inflammation in your airways.

- **Advanced glycation end products (AGEs).** These blood vessel-clogging compounds are found naturally in animal products and increase when the meat is cooked and processed. As they build up in your system, they contribute to lung inflammation. One study says that may be why eating meat is linked to breathing problems. Use an acidic marinade with a lemon or vinegar base on your meat to keep AGEs from forming when you cook.

- **Salt.** Since the '30s, studies have shown that high-salt diets increase asthma symptoms, but lowering the salt seems to decrease them.

How much is too much? A French study of nearly 1,000 participants over an average of seven years offers some insight. Those who ate more than three servings per week of cured meat like ham and sausage experienced worsening asthma symptoms over time. But for overall health benefits, experts at Harvard recommend limiting processed meats to once or twice a month.

No matter how you slice it, eating less processed meat may help reduce your asthma symptoms, but experts still caution you not to stop using your inhaler.

Catch your breath with the catch of the day

In the middle of an asthma attack, you might feel like a fish out of water. So would it sound fishy if someone told you to eat more salmon to ease your asthma symptoms? It's no fish tale. Salmon owes it all to two powerful nutrients.

Fight inflammation with omega-3 fatty acids. If you're like most Americans, you pile your plate with omega-6 fatty acids — fats found in foods like margarine and vegetable oil. While omega-6 has its benefits, it also has a downside — eating too much can promote inflammation and increase your risk for asthma.

Fortunately, you can balance out omega-6 by eating more omega-3 fatty acids found in fatty fish like salmon. Omega-3s, like eicosapentaenoic acid (EPA) and docosahexaenoic acid (DHA), help your body block omega-6 and fight the inflammation that can worsen asthma symptoms.

Because Americans eat up to 10 times more omega-6 fatty acids than omega-3s, being intentional about your diet is crucial. A 3.5-ounce serving of salmon is loaded with both EPA and DHA, so add it to your dinner plate to pump up the protection.

Decrease the severity of symptoms with vitamin D. Several clinical trials have reported that supplementing participants' usual asthma medication with vitamin D cut back on the need for corticosteroids during asthma attacks. Vitamin D supplements also lowered the risk of severe attacks that required an emergency room visit.

That 3.5-ounce salmon filet also boasts 13.3 micrograms (mcg) of vitamin D, which gets close to your daily requirement of 15 mcg if you're 70 and younger, or 20 mcg if you are over 70.

Steam up this mouthwatering meal to get more lung-boosting nutrients

How do you get the most sulforaphane from broccoli? Chop it up and wait 40 minutes before cooking. That releases the enzymes that create sulforaphane. You can also steam your greens to hang on to other nutrients. Cook it with salmon in one fell swoop using this easy method.

- Pull out your Dutch oven, steamer basket, aluminum foil, and two sheets of parchment paper.

- Add 1 inch of water to your Dutch oven. Wrap foil around the base of your metal steamer basket — or use a bamboo steamer basket — then set it on top of the water.

- Place your fish filets in a single layer on one piece of parchment. Season and garnish, then fold the paper to make a closed pouch.

- Place your broccoli on another piece of parchment. Fold it closed.

- Layer your two pouches in the steamer basket. Cover and cook over medium-high heat for about 10 minutes. Your fish will flake easily when done.

Save your money (and your health) when you make this swap

Have you noticed the upcharge for sodas and sweetened drinks at restaurants? A carbonated, sugary drink used to cost about 10 cents, but now you'll pay close to $3 for it. That's 30 times the cost of drinks 50 years ago.

The good news is you can still order water for free and drink all the refills you want. And skipping the sodas and sweetened drinks can mean better quality of life if you're living with asthma.

Pass over pop to keep your airways open. Sipping on sweetened drinks and sodas may make your asthma symptoms worse. Researchers in a recent study found that participants with asthma who drank soda seven or more times a week were more likely to have lower scores on their lung function tests compared to people who didn't drink them.

Fruit juices may seem like a tempting alternative, but look at the sugar content before you drink. Even without added sugars, fruit juices act more like sodas on your metabolism than whole fruit. But like sodas, they're often sweetened with high fructose corn syrup (HFCS).

Experts say HFCS may cause your lungs to shift into mucus-production gear. That can be bad news for asthma because excess mucus blocks your airways. Plus HFCS beverages have a high fructose-to-glucose ratio, which means there's no balance of glucose to help absorb the extra fructose. Researchers think the remaining fructose then helps create inflammatory substances that promote asthma.

Studies show that drinking these beverages just two to four times a week raises your risk for asthma, so look for drinks with no artificial sweeteners. Water is a great place to start.

Clear out those clogs in your pipes. Drinking water is part of a good asthma management plan because it hydrates your entire body. Here's how the right kind of hydration helps asthma.

- protects the linings of your airways and sinuses from drying out

- clears out mucus from your lungs

- helps control the level of histamines produced by your body

And as you drink to your health, you may want to stick to room temperature H2O. Refreshments that are too hot or too cold can cause your airways to narrow, leading to wheezing or coughing.

Breast cancer

Just for the health of it: Plant-based foods pack a powerful punch

What do creamy banana smoothies, roasted sweet potato fries, and zesty chili-lime salsa have in common? They're all part of a healthy, plant-based eating plan — one rich in fruits and vegetables — that may lower your chances of developing breast cancer. Here's how.

Beat back breast cancer with these nutrient-packed food staples. A California study of nearly 92,000 women between the ages of 22 and 84 found that participants who ate the most plant-based fare had a 15% lower chance of developing breast cancer than those who largely avoided eating fruits and vegetables.

Why? The researchers believe the insoluble fiber in plant-based foods may help lower your levels of estrogen — the hormone responsible for giving women female characteristics — by binding to and then carrying them out of your body. This may drop your risk of breast cancer because raised estrogen levels increase cell division. And the more your cells divide and multiply, the greater the opportunity for errors leading to cancer growth.

In addition, fruits and vegetables are high in cancer-fighting antioxidants and other powerful compounds. But they're just one part of this nutritious eating plan. Jazz up your meals by featuring these tasty — and filling — plant-based foods on your table.

- beans and legumes like chickpeas, pinto beans, lentils, peas, black beans, and peanuts

Eat
Tuna	Legumes
Whole grains	Green tea
Soy	Olive oil
Walnuts	

Avoid
Alcohol
Processed foods

- nuts and seeds like almonds, flaxseeds, walnuts, pistachios, sunflower seeds, and cashews

- whole grains like barley, popcorn, oats, brown rice, buckwheat, and bulgur

Skip the takeout to stay in shape. Of course, there's no food or diet that guarantees you won't get breast cancer. After all, things like genetics, age, and environmental factors play a part in promoting the disease.

But exchanging sodium- and sugar-heavy processed foods like bacon, fast food, and frozen pizza for healthier fare will help keep your weight in check, a key factor in keeping breast cancer at bay.

That's because being overweight or obese, just like smoking, opens the door to several types of cancer. British researchers found that to ring true after following the health of 163,000 postmenopausal women over eight years. The scientists discovered that the women who carried the most body fat were 70% more likely to develop breast cancer than the leanest women.

Experts think the reason might have to do with the late-in-life shift in estrogen production from the ovaries to fat cells. Excess body fat results in — you guessed it — the high estrogen levels that help cancer cells thrive.

Fight cancer with this 'D'elightful vitamin

Vitamin D is a must-have for seniors. Without it, your bones may become so brittle that a simple sneeze could result in a fracture. Need another reason to ensure you get enough of this nutrient? Well, it turns out that low levels of vitamin D may also increase your risk of developing breast cancer, especially if you're overweight.

That's according to a Brazilian study of some 600 postmenopausal women between the ages of 45 and 75 years old. Researchers found that women with breast cancer were more likely to have a vitamin D deficiency and be obese at the time of diagnosis than women in a control group who were cancer-free.

"Although published literature is inconsistent about the benefits of vitamin D levels and breast cancer, this study and others suggest that higher levels of vitamin D in the body are associated with lowered breast cancer risk," says Dr. JoAnn Pinkerton, executive director of The North American Menopause Society (NAMS). "Vitamin D may play a role in controlling breast cancer cells or stopping them from growing."

A study of more than 1,650 women with breast cancer found that those with high levels of vitamin D in their blood at the time of diagnosis had better long-term outcomes than those with low levels. It may be related to the vitamin's role in promoting the development of normal cells and the death of cancer cells.

NAMS published the research results in its journal *Menopause*.

Want to make sure you're getting enough of this nutrient each day? Seniors age 70 and younger should aim for 15 micrograms (mcg) each day. Those who are older should get 20 mcg daily. These foods pack a powerful punch when it comes to vitamin D.

Food	Amount	Micrograms
cod-liver oil	1 tablespoon	34
cooked swordfish	3 ounces	14
canned tuna, drained	3 ounces	4
fortified orange juice	1 cup	3.5
egg	1 large	1

Whip up a mouthwatering miso-walnut dressing

Think olive oil, walnuts, and miso — that fermented paste made from soybeans — make an odd trio? Think again. This Asian-inspired recipe combines all three into an incredibly creamy and healthy dressing that's sure to add a wow factor to your plate. Drizzle it over salads, vegetables, and even noodles.

To get started, you'll need these ingredients.

- 1/2 cup shelled walnuts
- 1/4 cup extra-virgin olive oil
- 2 tablespoons white miso paste
- 2 tablespoons white wine vinegar
- 1 teaspoon honey
- 1 medium clove of peeled garlic (optional)
- 1/4 cup warm water

Lightly toast a single layer of walnuts in a dry skillet at medium heat. Puree all the ingredients, adding the water a bit at a time, in a blender until smooth. Add salt to taste. Serve either warm or chilled.

3 superfoods that up your odds of staying in the pink

Way back in the 1920s American writer Victor Lindlahr proclaimed, "Ninety percent of the diseases known to man are caused by cheap foodstuffs. You are what you eat." His words still make sense today, considering your choice of foods can lower your risk of developing — and aid in the recovery — of chronic diseases like cancer.

So if you're looking to better your odds — 1 in 8 women will likely develop breast cancer in her lifetime — consider these tasty and often underrated superfoods.

Tap into the natural benefits of olive oil. People have been eating olive oil for thousands of years. But scientists only recently discovered that this liquid gold may keep breast cancer at bay.

That's according to Spanish researchers who followed almost 4,300 senior women for about five years. They found that those who added additional servings of extra-virgin olive oil to their Mediterranean diet — an eating plan featuring lots of fish, fruits, vegetables, and yes, olive oil — had a 62% lower risk of developing breast cancer than women who were simply advised to eat a low-fat diet.

> Spanish researchers recently found that women who ate supper at least two hours before bedtime had a 16% lower risk of developing breast cancer. The scientists say sleeping too soon after eating may negatively affect your ability to metabolize food, which could increase your risk of developing cancer.

Further research is needed, the scientists say, to confirm the results. But, they add, compounds in extra-virgin olive oil may help prevent damage to cellular DNA and put the brakes on tumor growth.

Crack a walnut for a wealth of health. Walnuts are tasty plain, toasted, or candied. And, it turns out, they may also curb the spread of breast cancer.

In a small recent study, women with breast cancer ate 2 ounces of walnuts — about 14 whole nuts — immediately following a biopsy and then daily until surgery about two weeks later. Researchers found that the genetic makeup of the women's tumors changed over the 14 days in ways that could slow the growth and hasten the death of breast cancer cells.

The scientists believe the results may be related to naturally occurring compounds — alpha linolenic acid, melatonin, beta-sitosterol, and vitamin E — in walnuts.

Arm yourself with soy's special powers. Soy-based foods are becoming popular replacements for meat and dairy products. And why not? They're high in vitamins, minerals, and fiber, and low in saturated fat. And soy may also increase the survival rates of women with certain types of breast cancer.

A nine-year study of more than 6,000 women with breast cancer found that those who ate the highest amount of soy — think miso, tofu, and soy yogurt — had a 21% lower risk of death from any cause than women who ate the least.

The decrease, however, occurred only in women whose cancer cells didn't need estrogen to grow and in women whose cancers weren't being treated with hormones. The researchers didn't provide a reason for their findings but believe they may be related to the high concentration of compounds called isoflavones in soybeans.

> Drinking alcoholic beverages raises a woman's risk of developing breast cancer. That's because alcohol can damage cells and increase levels of estrogen and other hormones linked to the disease. Your best bet? Limit yourself to one or two drinks a week or quit drinking alcohol altogether.

Green tea — an ancient drink steeped with cancer-crushing potential

Green tea may seem like all the rage these days. But the Chinese have long touted the health benefits of this light-bodied drink. In fact, practitioners of traditional medicine have used green tea for centuries to treat a wide range of ailments — from headaches and dizziness to heat stroke and poor digestion.

So what makes green tea so special? It's loaded with antioxidants called polyphenols that target and neutralize free radicals — unstable compounds that shamelessly attack and damage healthy cells. It's one of the reasons scientists say green tea may be effective in fighting many types of cancer and even boosting anti-cancer treatments.

In the case of breast cancer, it appears that the main polyphenol in green tea — a plant compound called epigallocatechin gallate, or EGCG for short — may hold promise in lowering the risk of developing the disease.

In one study, several hundred postmenopausal women supplemented their daily diets with decaffeinated green tea extract over the course of a year. The amount of extract was equal to five 8-ounce cups of brewed green tea each day. The women were between 50 and 70 years old and had dense breast tissue — lots of fibrous and glandular tissue compared with fat — that placed them at high risk for breast cancer. Here's what the researchers discovered.

- The older women in the study didn't experience any note-worthy change in the composition of their breast tissue. But those between the ages of 50 and 55 saw a significant decrease in density.

- Researchers say the effect was similar to that of tamoxifen, a drug used to reduce the risk of breast cancer.

Researchers aren't sure why green tea extract led to lower breast density in the younger group, but they do note that younger women have higher estrogen levels than their older counterparts. Because of that, they say, it makes sense that polyphenols targeting estrogen — a hormone that has been found to contribute to the formation of cancer cells — would have a greater effect on the younger women.

Of course, more research needs to be done on the promising health effects of green tea. But in the meantime, taste test this delicious and refreshing wonder food. It won't expand your waistline — just like water, green tea has absolutely no calories.

Cataracts

Sow the seeds of better vision with these cataract-crushing nutrients

Blurred vision caused by cataracts can wreck your golden years. These troublesome spots form when tissues within your eye's lens break down and clump together, forming cloudy patches.

More than half the people over age 65 have cataracts to some degree, mostly due to natural aging. But if you spend lots of time outdoors without sunglasses, the harmful ultraviolet light will boost your risk. Alcohol, smoking, and diabetes raise the chances of some types of cataracts, too.

Fortunately, you can help ward them off by tracking down foods loaded with these two vitamins and minerals.

Vitamin E can keep your sight sharp. Beefing up your vision could be as simple as getting enough vitamin E in your diet. A recent meta-analysis of 15,000 people found that those who got more of this nutrient were also the least likely to develop age-related cataracts.

A high-dose helping of this vitamin is also a part of the nutrient cocktail used in the AREDS supplement. Experts think it's so effective because it attacks free radicals before they get the chance to damage the lens of your eye.

Shoot for the daily recommendation of 15 milligrams (mg). You can get about halfway there from 3 1/2 tablespoons of sunflower seeds. Sprinkle them on oatmeal, salad, even your

Eat	
Sunflower seeds	Oranges
Orange juice	Spinach
Turmeric	Grapes
Red grape juice	Fatty fish
Pumpkin seeds	Flaxseed

Avoid

Alcohol
Sugary snacks and drinks

cooked vegetables, for a good dose of vitamin E throughout the day. Almonds and peanuts are great sources of vitamin E, too.

Call on this mighty mineral to keep your eyes clear. People with diabetes are at extra risk for eye problems. That's because excess blood sugar can damage your eye's lens.

But new animal studies suggest zinc could help save your vision. Researchers added this mineral to the diets of rats with diabetes-induced cataracts. Zinc slowed the progression of the cloudy spots by amping up the protective proteins and antioxidants in the lenses of their eyes.

Studies haven't been done on humans yet, so keep your ear to the ground for more information. In the meantime, experts say it's best to get around 11 mg of zinc for men or 8 mg for women every day. A 1-ounce serving of pumpkin seeds will get you 19% of your daily recommendation.

Pick up this special pumpkin seed year-round

Next time you're browsing nuts and seeds at the grocery stores, look for pepitas. They're the seeds from pumpkins, but not the big orange kind you carve up for Halloween.

Pepitas come from gourds bred specifically to grow shell-less seeds. Fortunately, they're just as healthy and full of zinc as the stuff you scoop out of your jack-o-lantern. And you don't have to wait until fall to get your hands on them.

Sprinkle a handful into your salads or stir them into soups to add a bit of crunch. Pepitas are also great baked into muffins, breads, or even cookies. Make sure to buy them unsalted so you don't overdo the sodium.

Wash down these powerful juices to protect your peepers

For centuries, sailors relied on the healing powers of citrus fruit to ward off the devastating effects of scurvy. Now experts think the vitamin C in these fruits could do more than prevent bleeding gums. It also holds the key to warding off cataracts.

Grab a glass of orange juice to "C" better. You might reach for some extra vitamin C when you're fighting off a cold, but your eyes could use a little bit of this power-packed nutrient, too.

A study published in the *International Journal of Ophthalmology* found that people with diets rich in vitamin C were less likely to get cataracts than people who didn't eat a lot of foods high in vitamin C. This nutrient helps fight off oxidative damage that can cause proteins to clump in the lens of your eye, contributing to cloudy vision and cataracts.

Boost your baby blues by making sure you get the recommended 75 to 90 milligrams of vitamin C a day. That's less than the amount you'll find in a cup of orange juice. You can also get loads of vitamin C from red peppers, broccoli, and grapefruit.

Go grape with a fantastic fruit drink to thwart cataracts. Red grape juice is chock-full of a chemical called resveratrol. And this plant compound offers up some powerful protection for your eyes.

Resveratrol boosts your body's production of its own naturally occurring antioxidant glutathione, which is important to your eye's lens. And it helps limit the formation of free radicals that can damage your eyes and lead to diseases like cataracts and glaucoma.

You can load up on resveratrol by drinking dark red grape juice. If you're worried about getting too much sugar from fruity drinks, eat whole grapes instead. Just look for grapes with dark red skins, because that's where the compound is most concentrated.

Is your daily supplement clouding your vision?

More isn't always better, especially when it comes to your diet. And while you may know the dangers of eating too much fat or sugar, you might not know that excess vitamin C can cause problems, too.

Even though this nutrient can be a sight-saver, research suggests long-term use of high-dose vitamin C supplements might actually increase your risk of cataracts. Researchers think super-high concentrations of vitamin C in the lens may contribute to oxidative stress that leads to tissue damage

A low-dose multivitamin will not put you at risk for cataracts, the study found. But if you're taking a high-dose vitamin C supplement, you could be getting more than 1,000% of your daily needs, which is a problem.

Instead of reaching for megadose supplements, stick with natural sources like oranges and grapefruit to meet your daily vitamin C requirement of 75 to 90 milligrams, unless your doctor recommends otherwise.

Sup on spinach to steer clear of cataracts

Did you know spinach can be used to diffuse explosives? Seriously — scientists discovered that enzymes derived from the leafy green veggie can actually turn TNT into carbon dioxide and water. So it may not be so hard to believe that spinach could stop age-related cataracts in their tracks.

Spinach is packed with this sight-saving dynamic duo. When it comes to protection for your eyes, you can't top lutein and zeaxanthin. These two phytochemicals are rock stars at warding off oxidative damage.

A review of studies proved just how powerful they are. Scientists found that people who ate the foods highest in lutein and zeaxanthin were 23% less likely to develop nuclear cataracts. This is the most common type caused by the gradual hardening and yellowing of the lens.

Even better? It only takes as little as 4 milligrams a day to slow the progression of cataracts. You'll get five times that in a single cup of cooked spinach.

This vital vitamin will help you dodge clouded vision. According to a recent study conducted in Spain, vitamin K could also help ward off age-related cataracts.

Researchers examined the eyes and the diets of 1,900 people over 5 1/2 years. They found that those who ate foods rich in this powerful nutrient were less likely to need cataract surgery than people who didn't get enough vitamin K.

Why? The scientists think it comes down to two things. First, vitamin K can act as an antioxidant, protecting you from the cell damage that causes cloudy vision. And it also helps lower sugar concentrations in your blood and in your eye's lens, which can help prevent cataracts from forming.

Men should aim for about 120 micrograms (mcg) of vitamin K every day, and women should try to get around 90 mcg. Fortunately, cooked spinach clocks in at a whopping 889 mcg per cup.

Call on turmeric to spice up your sight

Your spice rack does more than zest up your dinner plate. If you know what to look for, you'll find potent protection against all sorts of ailments. And one exotic ingredient could hold the key to thwarting cataracts.

Turmeric — a golden spice from India — is loaded with a naturally occurring chemical called curcumin. And experts say this nutrient has some serious sight-saving powers.

Studies show it can fight off oxidative damage to your eye's lens. And it helps pump up the levels of vitamin C in your eyes as well, so you'll get a double dose of antioxidants.

Researchers haven't figured out how much turmeric you need to add to your diet to fight cataracts, but keep your eyes peeled for more information in the future.

In the meantime, sprinkle this exotic spice on roast veggies, stir it into your morning scrambled eggs, or add it to a smoothie. It's a good idea to add black or cayenne pepper to your turmeric, too. It will help your body absorb more sight-saving antioxidants.

Fish or flax: How to choose the best omega-3 for you

You know that omega-3 fatty acids are an important part of a healthy diet. After all, studies show that getting more of these fantastic fats are a surefire way to lower your risk of cataracts. Experts say they boost the levels of good HDL cholesterol in your body. That means more antioxidants, like vitamin E, are ferried to your eyes where they can protect you from oxidative damage.

But there's more than one way to get omega-3s in your diet. And they're not all created equal.

- Fatty fish. Animal sources of omega-3, like salmon and sardines, are largely made up of long-chain omega-3 fatty acids called eicosapentaenoic acid (EPA) and docosahexaenoic acid (DHA). These are easily absorbed and used by your body.

- Flaxseeds. Plant-based omega-3s aren't the same as the ones you'll get from fish. Instead, you'll get a short-chain fatty acid, known as alpha linolenic acid (ALA). Before your body can use it, ALA needs to be broken down into EPA and DHA. Unfortunately, only a small percentage of ALA is converted into usable fats.

Plant-based omega-3 fatty acid doesn't quite measure up to the protection you'll find in fish. However, if you're a vegetarian or allergic to seafood, it's still a good alternative.

Cavities

TEAmwork: Win the battle against bacteria

Tea isn't just a soothing drink, it's a fighter against cavity-causing bacteria. And if you choose to pump yours up with ginger, lemon, or honey, your teeth could be in for an even greater victory.

If you've never had a cavity, consider yourself lucky. This bothersome problem starts with a sticky film called plaque building up on your teeth. When bacteria in the plaque ferment the food you eat, they produce acids that break down tooth enamel. You can help prevent this decay by brushing and flossing regularly and also by eating right.

Green tea is one way to help. It's packed with polyphenols that can stop leading cavity culprits *Streptococcus mutans (S. mutans)* and *Candida albicans* in their tracks. These bacteria cause even greater damage when they partner up, so ending their spread is key.

One of green tea's prime defenders is the polyphenol epigallocatechin-3-gallate (EGCG). It stops bacteria growth and may even help with tooth sensitivity. Want to give your tea even more of a boost? These three tooth-savers are perfect cavity-fighting additions.

Ginger provides a one-two punch.
This spice is known to be both anti-inflammatory and antimicrobial. But it's ginger's bacteria-fighting ability that takes center stage in your mouth. Research has found it can curb unwanted *S. mutans* growth on your tooth's enamel. Add some ground or sliced ginger to your tea to double up on cavity prevention.

Eat	
Grapes	Green tea
Ginger	Garlic
Cloves	Milk

Avoid

Sugary cereals

Soy and other sweetened milks

Frozen juices

Acidic foods and drinks

Turn your favorites into a cavity-fighting tea

If you love the flavors of ginger, honey, and lemon, why not use them to make their own cavity-fighting tea? As an added benefit, it fights colds, too. Try this simple recipe.

Slice 2 inches of fresh ginger, and combine with 4 cups of water in a saucepan. Bring to a boil, then lower the heat, and cover the pan. Allow it to simmer five to 10 minutes, or leave it longer for a spicier drink. Remove from the heat and take out the ginger slices. Add 3 tablespoons of lemon juice and 4 tablespoons of honey, and stir until dissolved.

This tea will make four servings. Refrigerate any leftovers, and reheat as needed.

Lemon gives cavities a sucker punch. If you're in the mood for citrus, lemon is a good choice. It contains potent antioxidants, and when tested against *S. mutans*, it shows antibacterial qualities, too.

Adding a slice of lemon to your tea may be just what the dentist ordered. Don't let its zing zap your teeth's strength, though. An overly acidic mouth can wear away your bite, so use lemon prudently.

Honey is a sweet alternative. You don't have to put your teeth's health on the line when you sweeten your tea. Just use honey.

Honey is made up of the sugars fructose and glucose. It has less of both than the white sugar you're used to, but is sweeter because of its extra fructose. That helps you use less, which in the long run, may help ward off cavities.

Honey's antibacterial qualities also make it a good choice. Research has shown it reduces the acids that threaten your teeth and keeps bad bacteria from building up. A recent study found that manuka, a honey from New Zealand, is particularly effective at stopping *S. mutans*.

Scientists have discovered that bacteria don't build up a resistance to honey, so you'll benefit from using it long term. Look for manuka honey online.

Enjoy a 'grape' new way to avoid cavities

Not everyone can be fed grapes off gold trays like movie royalty. But no matter how you eat them, you'll benefit from their cavity-defying virtues. Whether dried into raisins or eaten fresh off the vine, grapes are ready to pass on their "mouth"watering protection.

Raisins shake off reputation as a cavity causer. Let's face it, raisins are sweet and sticky. And that's not great for your teeth. Because of this, some experts have warned people not to eat them. But the truth is, these sweet little nuggets are not as bad as they seem.

The three major contributors to cavities are food clinging to your teeth, an acidic mouth, and the presence of bad bacteria. Raisins may surprise you by how well they avoid these pitfalls.

* In one test, participants tasted different snacks and labeled raisins equally as gummy as chewy snacks like granola bars. But surprisingly, people cleared the raisins from their teeth fairly quickly, which means they're less likely to cause cavities.

* A low pH in your mouth means it's acidic. That's dangerous because the acid eats away at enamel. In a study on children and raisin cereal, raisins never dropped the pH to a dangerous level. In fact, scientists think raisins may

> Avoid brushing your teeth right after you eat or drink something acidic, like orange juice. You may think you're cleaning it off your teeth, but your weakened enamel is more likely to be damaged. Instead, rinse your mouth with water right after, and wait at least 30 minutes to an hour before heading in with a toothbrush.

actually help clear out acidic foods that are more likely to cause damage.

- Raisins fight *Streptococcus mutans (S. mutans)*, one of the bacteria most associated with cavities. Some experts think raisins combat these bad guys through compounds that stop bacterial growth. Others suggest it may be their antioxidants at work.

The bottom line? Although raisins are sweet and sticky, studies show they don't stick to your teeth long enough to cause cavities and may help clear other sugars from your mouth. So don't be afraid to enjoy them as a healthy snack.

Your tooth-saver may start on a stem. You probably know that wine has been touted for certain health benefits. That's because grapes are filled with antioxidant power from stem to seed.

Polyphenols are a type of phyto-chemical, and the ones found in red wine grapes may help protect your teeth. For example, caffeic acid has shown antimicrobial activity against *S. mutans* and other bacteria during lab testing. One reason may be because it creates compounds that produce hydrogen peroxide, which damages bacterial DNA.

> Grapeseed extract may extend the life of your filling. It strengthens the layer of your teeth called dentin, where resin fillings attach. That helps create a better seal between the two and prevent future damage. Scientists are working on putting this exciting new research into practice.

Grapes are also bursting with flavonoids like catechin and epicatechin. A recent study shows that these two may protect your pearly whites by keeping bacteria from sticking.

But you don't have to reach for a glass of wine to get these bacteria-blasting phytochemicals. Try munching on a cup of juicy red grapes to take advantage of their cavity-fighting nutrients.

The frozen treat that can ruin your teeth

Summertime heat got you longing for an ice-cold popsicle? Before you reach for a chilly treat, consider how long it takes you to eat it.

Frozen juices like popsicles can be dangerous to your teeth because they linger in your mouth. That gives acids more time to wear away your enamel.

See how your snack compares to similar options.

- Regular fruit juice is also risky for your teeth. It contains sugars and acids that can erode your teeth and create a cavity-friendly environment.

  Experts recommend drinking juice through a straw and rinsing your mouth with water afterward to help protect your teeth.

- Whole fruits can be high in sugar and acids, but they bring other benefits like fiber. It's best to choose low-sugar and low-acid fruits like peaches and berries over more risky options like pineapple.

The worst breakfast for your teeth — and how to fix it

Cereal is the perfect option for a quick and easy breakfast. But not every bowlful is created equal, and if you're not careful you could damage your teeth in surprising ways.

Close the box lid on candy-like cereal. Sugary cereals may be tasty, but they're one of the worst foods you can eat for breakfast. That's because cereal provides the perfect combination of refined sugar and starch that bacteria love to feed on. And when they do, they produce acid that can erode the enamel on your teeth.

Your tooth enamel starts to lose minerals around a pH of 5.5. Any pH under 7 is acidic, and the lower it goes the more acidic — and cavity-prone — it becomes.

The sugar content of your favorite sweet breakfast could push you into the danger zone after only one bowl. An easy fix is to pick a new, healthier cereal like General Mills' Fiber One or Kellogg's Puffed Wheat. They both have a high-fiber and low-sugar content.

Your milk choice matters, too. Alternatives to cow's milk are trendy, but watch out for soy milk. Surprisingly, it could increase your risk for cavities.

> If you love cereal but want to protect your teeth, your best option may be to eat your cereal dry, then enjoy a glass of milk. Drinking milk afterward, rather than mixed in, reduces the acid caused by eating the sugary cereal and keeps your mouth pH in a safe zone.

- One study found that participants who drank soy milk for 15 days showed a loss of minerals in their enamel while those who drank cow's milk showed an increase. Researchers believe soy milk is a greater cavity risk because of its added sugar. Plus your body has a harder time absorbing the calcium in soy milk.

- In another study, plaque grew the most with soy milk compared to cow and almond milks. And soy milk was least likely to keep mouth pH from plunging into the acid zone.

Classic cow's milk is a great choice if you like it. It's one of the best at controlling acid levels in your mouth and has other health benefits like calcium and phosphate.

If you prefer to stick to a substitute, almond milk is your best bet. But go with an unsweetened option. It causes less plaque than sweetened almond, soy, and cow's milk. And it won't create an acidic environment like sweetened almond milk will.

2 flavorful spices that fight cavities

The next time you bake ham for dinner, cover it with whole cloves. Making your family's favorite Italian dish? Include plenty of garlic. These potent ingredients not only add flavor, they help protect your teeth.

- Garlic outperforms other foods when pitted against the bacterium *S. mutans*. This is partly because of allicin, its main compound, which is released when you crush or chop a garlic clove. Allicin has antibacterial properties.

  In one study, researchers found garlic was even more effective than honey, lemon, and ginger at stopping the cavity-creating bacteria.

- The spicy warmth of cloves is the perfect addition to fall and winter recipes. Their warm flavor isn't their only benefit, though.

  In a study published by the *Journal of Clinical and Diagnostic Research*, clove oil's antimicrobial properties outdid products like tea tree oil and neem at warding off *S. mutans*.

Chronic pain

Fight persistent pain with the help of powerful vitamins

If you've ever smacked your finger with a hammer, you know it smarts. But that kind of pain usually goes away after a while. Chronic pain, on the other hand, lasts more than three months or beyond the expected time for healing.

What do both types of pain have in common? Researchers say the origin is inflammation.

Unfortunately, some say chronic inflammation is part of aging and even call it "inflammaging." But that doesn't mean constant aches are inevitable. Choose foods rich in vitamins to start shutting down the inflammatory cycle that contributes to chronic pain.

Boost your body's pain-fighting potential with antioxidants. Everyday living adds stress to your cells. As you digest food, for example, your body produces free radicals — unstable molecules that lack one electron. Because they are unbalanced, these free radicals travel through your body, like a band of pickpockets, trying to steal electrons from stable, healthy cells. When they succeed, they cause cell damage, called oxidation.

Over time free radicals can build up, further damaging already-injured tissue and causing inflammation, which can lead to chronic pain in muscles, tissues, and joints.

Eat

Black pepper	Carrots
Cayenne	Chickpeas
Ginger	Kiwi
Oregano	Red peppers
Strawberries	Tangerines
Turmeric	Yogurt

Avoid

Gluten-containing products if sensitive to ATIs

High-FODMAP foods during elimination period

Luckily, you can help the damage with antioxidants. They fight oxidation by combining with free radicals, or giving them an electron, to make them stable. Your body produces some antioxidants itself, but you can also get loads of them from fresh fruits and vegetables in the form of vitamins A, E, and C.

Head off hurts with a tasty roasted carrot hummus

How do you pack a world record into one snack? You make a 10-ton batch of hummus like they did in Lebanon in 2010. It held enough pain-fighting, inflammation-busting vitamins to have the city dancing a jig. Make yours with yogurt and carrots for an extra blast of nutrients. Here's how.

Soak 6 ounces of dried chickpeas overnight. Rinse and boil for an hour. While they're cooking, toss 1 cup of baby carrots in extra-virgin olive oil and balsamic vinegar. Roast the carrots on high until tender, around 45 minutes. Now you're ready to put your hummus together.

- Puree two to four garlic cloves with 3 tablespoons of lemon juice.

- Add the chickpeas, along with 1/4 cup of the water you cooked them in. Add the carrots, and blend until creamy.

- Add salt to taste, 4 tablespoons extra-virgin olive oil, a teaspoon ground cumin, and 1/4 cup of plain Greek yogurt. Blend until smooth.

Help yourself to this vitamin-packed pair. Sneak some variety into your snacking routine by combining fruits and veggies in creative ways to deliver an antioxidant punch.

Delicious red peppers are a great place to start. They're rich in vitamins A and E. Plus just one pepper delivers more than 100% of your daily vitamin C, a nutrient that has recently been studied in supplement form with good results for relieving certain types of chronic pain.

Next, dip those sliced peppers in a creamy hummus. Animal studies show B vitamins play a big role in blocking pain intensity. And the main ingredients in hummus — chickpeas — are high in B6 and thiamine (B1). Plus if you make it with yogurt instead of tahini, you'll also get vitamin B12. Being too low in this nutrient is linked to peripheral neuropathy, nerve damage that causes pain and numbness.

Spice up your salad and entree to tackle your pain

Spices and pain share some things in common. Both can be edgy and sharp. But while pain adds an unpleasant kick to your life, the compounds in certain seasonings can calm pain from inflammation.

Turmeric, ginger, oregano, cayenne, paprika, and black pepper are all loaded with potent pain-fighters. While that doesn't guarantee they'll zap all your pain, they are sure to tickle your taste buds and liven up your supper plans along the way.

Dress your salad for pain-fighting success. Zesty salads add zing to your meal, so be sure yours pops with an olive oil and yogurt dressing seasoned by turmeric, black pepper, and fresh ginger. Why? These spices sport antioxidant and anti-inflammatory properties.

Turmeric's active ingredient is a polyphenol called curcumin. In a recent review of eight randomized clinical trials, experts looked at curcumin's ability to cut back on pain in a number of conditions ranging from arthritis to acute muscle injury. The result? Curcumin supplementation significantly reduced pain.

Pair turmeric with black pepper to get the full benefit. Piperine — a compound in black pepper — increases the rate of curcumin absorption by 2,000%. That's nothing to sneeze at.

Although data on ginger's pain-relieving potential is limited, research points to its ability to block two nasty compounds — prostaglandins and leukotrienes. Both are linked to inflammation, swelling, and pain.

Punch back pain with a lively Moroccan chicken entree.
Transport yourself to "the farthest land of the setting sun" with a
Moroccan chicken stew. Hints of turmeric, ginger, pepper, oregano,
cayenne, and paprika flirt boldly with tender zucchini, garlic,
onion, celery, tomatoes, chickpeas, and chicken. It's a kaleido-
scope of flavors that may be
more comforting than your
grandma's chicken soup.

Take oregano, for example. It's
loaded with beta-caryophyllene,
a chemical that may help relieve
pain associated with inflammation and nerve damage.

Next, that pinch of cayenne
and dash of paprika — the
hot varieties — you toss into
your stew also protect against
pain and inflammation. Both

> Weakness, muscle stiffness,
> and cramps are hard to ignore.
> These symptoms can flare up
> when you're low in potassium,
> an electrolyte involved in
> nerve and muscle activity. You
> can lose potassium from
> chronic vomiting and diarrhea,
> and from medications that
> increase urination. Up your
> potassium levels with a delicious
> fruit salad of tangerines, kiwi,
> cantaloupe, and strawberries.

spices contain capsaicin, a compound that lowers the amount of
pain messages that make it from your nerves to your brain.

2 proven plans to deep-six fibromyalgia aches

Got bananas, carrots, and strawberries? This trio of foods might
be among the best to pit against the trio of pain symptoms —
tenderness, chronic aches, and deep muscle pain — common to
fibromyalgia (FM). Here's why you might want to blend them
together with some cold water for your next smoothie.

They're part of a raw vegetarian diet. An observational study
back in 2001 suggested that people with FM could benefit from
loading up on fruits and veggies and avoiding meat. Each day for
seven months, participants drank about 2 to 4 cups of carrot juice
and ate leafy salads and fruit while following a mostly raw vegetarian

diet. By the end of the study, they were experiencing better flexibility as well as less pain and a wider range of motion in their shoulders.

Fast forward to 2019. A large review continues to recommend a vegetarian diet for FM pain. Scientists aren't sure why raw fruits and vegetables help FM pain but say it may be because they boost antioxidant levels in your body and fight inflammation.

They're part of a low-FODMAP diet. You've probably heard of a low-FODMAP (fermentable oligosaccharides, disaccharides, monosaccharides, and polyols) diet for digestive problems because it restricts carbs that are known to trigger bloating, gas, and stomach pain. Did you know it may also help with fibromyalgia symptoms?

Participants in a clinical trial followed a strict diet to cut back on FODMAPs for four weeks, then reintroduced some FODMAPs back into their diet for four more weeks. They found that their fibromyalgia pain was reduced when they followed this plan.

Reduce	Replace with
lactose in dairy	lactose-free alternatives
fructose-rich foods like apples, mangoes, pears, watermelon, honey, sweeteners	bananas, blueberries, grapes, melons, oranges, strawberries
fructan-rich foods like wheat, rye, onions, garlic	corn, spelt, rice, oat, gluten-free products
galactan-rich foods like cabbage, chickpeas, beans, lentils	carrots, celery, green beans, lettuce, pumpkin, tomatoes, potatoes
polyol-rich foods like apricots, cherries, nectarines, plums, cauliflower	grapefruit, kiwi, lemons, limes, passion fruit

FM symptoms seem to be linked to the makeup of your intestinal bacteria. A short-term low-FODMAP diet may help you balance your gut bacteria, which can cut down on inflammation that's associated with pain.

Go against the grain of pain with a gluten-free diet

No doubt you've heard gluten causes problems for people with celiac disease (CD). But what if proteins in gluten-containing food are causing pain in your joints, muscles, head, and stomach even when you don't have CD?

Unless labeled "gluten free," your breakfast cereal, bread, and pasta contain gluten. And all gluten products contain proteins called ATIs (amylase trypsin inhibitors). According to researchers, these ATIs could be the secret culprit of some people's pain, rather than the gluten itself.

ATI proteins provoke your immune system. "As well as contributing to the development of bowel-related inflammatory conditions, we believe that ATIs can promote inflammation of other immune-related chronic conditions outside of the bowel," says Professor Detlef Schuppan, lead researcher of a recent study that links ATIs to chronic health conditions.

"ATIs from wheat activate specific types of immune cells in the gut and other tissues, thereby potentially worsening the symptoms of preexisting inflammatory illnesses," says Schuppan. That may include conditions like rheumatoid arthritis, multiple sclerosis, lupus, and inflammatory bowel disease — all known to cause pain.

Go gluten free to see if you have less pain. Gluten-free diets have already been linked to pain reduction in people with neuropathy caused by gluten sensitivity. And researchers hope they'll soon have enough studies to recommend an ATI-free diet for folks with certain conditions. In the meantime, you can still talk to your doctor about avoiding these grains. Be on the lookout for them in your flour and processed foods.

- oats (unless labeled "gluten free")
- rye
- triticale (wheat and rye crossed)
- barley
- wheat (including modern varieties like durum)

Your doctor may suggest you avoid these grains for a while to see if symptoms improve. Then you can slowly add them back in, starting with older wheat varieties that have shown less ATI immune activity like einkorn, emmer (farro), and spelt. If your pain level doesn't increase when you reintroduce certain foods, you may be able to eat them consistently so you can get fiber, vitamins, and other nutrients into your diet more easily.

On the horizon: Calm your nerve pain with natural supplements

Are constant aches getting on your nerves? Good news — the latest research says supplements show promise for fighting off the tingling, numbness, and shooting pain associated with nerve damage.

Melatonin puts the ZZZs on pain. Melatonin is best known for controlling your sleep cycle, but new research suggests this hormone is doing anything but snoozing inside your cells. Based on several studies, researchers have a few theories about how melatonin supplements help heal nerve damage.

- Melatonin may act as an antioxidant, preventing free radical damage and protecting nerves in your peripheral nervous system, the ones outside your brain and spinal cord.

- It may also lessen scar formation following nerve injury in a number of ways, including blocking collagen production. Without the scarring, nerves can heal faster.

When combined with other therapy, melatonin also shows potential to relieve headaches, chronic back pain, abdominal pain, and sleep disorders associated with fibromyalgia.

While it's still early and dosage limits need to be decided by more advanced trials, this sleepy supplement may yet prove to be a wake-up call for chronic pain relief.

ALC offers TLC for painful peripheral neuropathy

A brand-new review published in the *Journal of Pain Research* has some good news. Acetyl-L-carnitine (ALC), a supplement form of the amino acid L-carnitine, is safe and effective for lowering pain intensity in people with peripheral neuropathy. The meta-analysis of four randomized controlled trials says the supplement promotes healing in damaged nerve fibers.

To find out more about this painful condition and how ALC can help people with high blood sugar, check out *Stop diabetes from getting on your nerves with ALC* in the *Diabetes* chapter.

Protect against pain with procyanidins. These antioxidants are flavonoids found in foods like chocolate, apples, and cranberry juice. Often used in the form of grapeseed extract, researchers praise them for reducing gut discomfort and relieving the pain and swelling associated with gout.

And they seem to be a rising star for neuropathic pain. This type of pain — caused by injury, vitamin deficiencies, and conditions like diabetes — stems from damage to nerves that carry messages to your brain and spinal cord.

According to a recent animal study published in the *Journal of Neuroinflammation*, procyanidins help block enzymes and proteins that cause pain and inflammation. Other animal studies suggest they also support the myelin sheath, the fatty sleeve that surrounds and protects your nerves.

While you can buy grapeseed extract supplements in stores and online, more research needs to be done before they get the green light for your nerve pain.

Colds & Flu

Mission critical — stop flu virus with this secret weapon

Your body is primed and ready to fight off all kinds of attacks. But the flu virus is like a ninja — cloaked in a special protein that lets it slip into your cells before your immune system knows it's there.

Fortunately, you can call on a secret agent to break up mucus, open sinuses, and fight germs — tea. The best part? It's made from three pantry staples.

- Green tea. It's loaded with catechins, phytochemicals that barricade influenza's entry into cells. In one study, children who drank 1 to 5 cups of green tea daily cut their risk of getting the flu. In another study, researchers gave adults green tea capsules equaling 10 cups of tea daily for three months. Fewer got sick compared to the placebo group, and those who did weren't sick as long.

- Honey. Nerve fibers that trigger cough are near the nerve fibers that help you taste sweetness. Researchers think these may interact when you eat honey and give you an advantage in subduing a rogue cough. And honey's got the World Health Organization's approval for this mission. To get more antioxidants, go with the darker varieties.

- Turmeric. Call in this powerful condiment to elude the flu. Turmeric's curcumin — an antioxidant-of-all-trades — fights several viral, bacterial, and fungal foes, including influenza in one test tube study.

Eat

Elderberries	Honey
Turmeric	Green tea
Garlic	Winter squash
Beans	Mushrooms
Nutritional yeast	
Vitamin D-fortified cereal	

Avoid

Processed snacks like chips and crackers

Here are two ways to secure the benefits of honey turmeric green tea.

Prepare it hot to soothe sinuses. Brew your tea for four minutes on low heat, around 167 degrees. The low temp will help preserve the catechins and flavor. For each cup, stir in up to 1/4 teaspoon of ground, grated, or powdered turmeric, and add honey to taste. Then breathe in the steam and drink it warm to let the water vapor tickle your irritated sinuses and stimulate mucus flow.

Mucus cleans and protects your sinuses. It thickens when you're sick, which can make you more miserable. Because bacteria cling to mucus, encouraging your nose to run means you get rid of both faster.

Cool it to take out more germs. To get even more flu-fighting compounds, steep 4 teaspoons of loose tea leaves or three tea bags in a quart of water in the refrigerator for 12 hours.

A study of brewing methods revealed a higher level of antioxidants from this cold-brew technique for two reasons. First, the tea leaves are in the water longer, allowing more of the good compounds to infuse the drink. Second, the low temperature protects the beneficial compounds that can break down in higher temps.

Don't want to wait? Brewing tea over low heat for five minutes then quickly icing it is nearly as effective as the cold-brew method. The rapid cooling protects compounds from long exposure to harsh, high temperatures. Plus you can stir in the honey when it's still warm to help it dissolve easier.

Thwart cold and flu viruses with a fabled berry

Legend has it an elder tree can protect you from a lightning strike. While there's no proof to back up that folklore, research shows more promise for the elder tree's medicinal powers. It may not shield you from a bolt of electricity, but its berries could protect you when cold and flu season strikes.

Set up a roadblock for the flu virus — naturally. A new test tube study found that elderberry extract works on several levels to shut down influenza. How? Phytochemicals — natural plant compounds — in elderberries help block the flu virus from infecting cells. They can also jump-start the immune response and stop the virus from reproducing inside infected cells.

Are your snacks weakening your flu vaccine?

According to researchers at Michigan State University, a common food additive called tert-butylhydroquinone, or tBHQ, may make your flu vaccine less effective. This ingredient — found in cooking oils, frozen meats, and processed foods — helps stabilize fats. But it's not always on the food label.

In the study, flu-infected mice ate either a diet containing tBHQ or a control diet. Researchers saw a drop in the number of cells that could identify the flu in the tBHQ group.

"It's important for the body to be able to recognize a virus and remember how to effectively fight it off," says Robert Freeborn, co-leader of the study. "That's the whole point of vaccines, to spur this memory and produce immunity. TBHQ seems to impair this process."

Experts believe you could be eating as much as 1,100% of the acceptable daily intake of tBHQ. Cutting down on processed snacks will limit the amount of tBHQ that sneaks into your diet.

An uncommon solution to cut down a cold. In a recent clinical trial, researchers gave 312 airline passengers elderberry extract for 10 days prior to taking a lengthy overseas flight. Participants continued the supplements five days into their trip. On average, the elderberry group recovered from their colds two days faster than the control group. Plus their symptoms weren't as severe.

Once again, researchers point to phytochemicals as the reason behind the health benefits, this time emphasizing their antioxidant activity.

Participants took 600 to 900 milligrams of elderberry extract daily, but you can also get a heap of antioxidants from the berries themselves. You'll generally find them dried in stores and online. If you do get your hands on raw berries, cook them before serving.

Raw elderberries can make you sick. Luckily, research shows that boiling the berries for around 10 minutes doesn't break down the beneficial compounds.

Elderberry syrup — sweeten your respiratory relief

Homemade elderberry syrup livens up pancakes and ice cream. Freeze it for popsicles or mix it into a salad vinaigrette. Some folks even take it by the spoonful for a daily immune boost.

Make your own elderberry syrup for just over $12, which is half the cost of buying it — and you control the ingredients. It's easy to whip up a 16-ounce batch.

Just bring 1 cup of dried elderberries, 1/2 teaspoon of ground cloves, and 4 cups of water to a boil. If desired, add a teaspoon of cinnamon and a tablespoon of ginger. Then cover and simmer for up to an hour.

Next, mash the berries and strain the mixture. Allow to cool, then stir in a cup of honey. Store in the refrigerator in an air-tight container.

Elderberries kick-start your immune response, so they may interfere with immune suppression medications. Talk to your doctor if you're concerned about drug interactions.

Soup up your fight against germs

A cold or flu can make you want to crawl back under your covers and hide for days. Whether you're already sick or trying to avoid it, a hot, comforting soup loaded with tasty virus-fighting vegetables may go a long way toward helping you feel better and stay well.

Soothe cold symptoms with a fiery broth. The Centers for Disease Control and Prevention recommends you drink plenty of fluids when you're sick. Why? Fevers, medications, mucus production — these can quickly dry you out. And severe dehydration can be dangerous. Sipping on a hearty soup broth is a surefire way to stay hydrated.

Sprinkle in some cayenne pepper to loosen up the mucus in your nose and head. About 1/8 to 1/4 of a teaspoon is a good place to start for a pot of soup. Feeling achy? That spunky little spice has capsaicin in it, which is known to be a pain reliever.

Researchers haven't recommend a dose for soothing symptoms, but people have used capsaicin-packed chili peppers in traditional medicine for coughs, sore throats, and aches.

Fiber-filled veggies fend off the flu. Researchers recently discovered a high-fiber diet protects animals from the flu virus. They believe the reason has to do with fiber's ability to enhance the part of the immune system responsible for stopping and getting rid of viruses.

While research is still in the early phases, it won't hurt to stock your broth with these high-fiber ingredients.

- winter squash
- celery
- beans
- mushrooms
- potatoes
- onions
- carrots

Cook up a cup of each of these vegetables in about 2 quarts of broth. Then chop a clove of garlic and add it to your simmering soup with a tablespoon of dried rosemary. A serving of this tasty medley, containing a cup of the mixed veggies, offers more than 17% of your daily recommendation of fiber and may add a measure of flu prevention to your day.

Drop a little nutritional yeast into your soup to boost the flavor and your immune defenses. In one study during the intense months of cold season, participants who took 450 milligrams of yeast beta glucan fiber twice daily — equal to about a spoonful of nutritional yeast — for 26 weeks had significantly fewer infections than the placebo group.

Block the cough, sniffle, and sneeze with vitamin D

About 10% of emergency room visits in the U.S. result from acute respiratory infections. Many are caused by the common cold, bronchitis, or pneumonia. Fortunately, you can protect your upper respiratory assets by stepping up your vitamin D game.

Drop your risk of respiratory infections with supplements. Some researchers believe vitamin D helps by supporting your immune response to certain bacteria and viruses.

A review of 25 randomized controlled trials published in the leading medical journal *The BMJ* suggests vitamin D can lower the risk of acute respiratory infections when taken in daily or weekly doses ranging from 7.5 to 100 micrograms (mcg).

"The protective effects of vitamin D supplementation are strongest in those who have the lowest vitamin D levels, and when supplementation is given daily or weekly rather than in more widely spaced doses," says lead researcher Professor Adrian Martineau.

In fact, the risk of getting a respiratory infection dropped by nearly half in those individuals. Ask your doctor if a vitamin D supplement is right for you.

Upping your virus "D"-fense is easy at breakfast. If you're under 70 you need 15 mcg of vitamin D daily, or 20 mcg daily if you're older. Many nutritionists recommend you get as much D from your food as possible, so supplements should only be reinforcements.

Next time you're at the grocery store, plan your breakfast of champions by checking food labels for vitamin D fortification. The nutrient is often added to cereal, milk, orange juice, and yogurt, but it occurs naturally in egg yolks and cheese.

Triumph over a cold may be near with olive leaf extract

Ancient Greeks massaged their Olympians with olive oil for wisdom and strength. Winners of the games earned an olive leaf crown. Today, athletes have put olive leaves to another use — bouncing back after a cold.

In a recent study in *Nutrients*, researchers asked a small group of high school athletes to take either 20 grams of olive leaf extract (OLE) supplements or a placebo for nine weeks. The result? OLE didn't prevent illness, but cut the number of sick days by 28%.

How does it work? Olive leaf contains oleuropein and hydroxytyrosol, two polyphenols known to have antiviral and antioxidant properties. Researchers suspect OLE may stop the virus from reproducing, which then improves your body's defense.

Researchers see promise in this ancient extract, but it's still early. Although you can find OLE on the market, ask your doctor before starting the supplement.

Clear out a cold faster with these classic remedies

It's inevitable. The common cold barrels in like a freight train every year. If you catch it, should you load up on vitamin C and zinc to get rid of it as quickly as possible? Experts continue to debate their cold-fighting capabilities. So what's the latest word?

To supplement or not to supplement? Good question. Vitamin C and zinc both support your immune system, but that doesn't mean taking pills every day will keep you from getting sick.

Recent research published in the *Cochrane Database of Systematic Reviews* found that taking at least 1 gram (g) of vitamin C daily shortened the length of adults' colds by about half a day and improved symptom severity. Researchers also reported that taking 8 g on a single day shortened colds even more.

Likewise, zinc lozenges may limit the amount of time you're sick — possibly up to 33%. A recent meta-analysis suggests a dose of 80 milligrams a day could be effective if the lozenges don't contain citric acid, which binds zinc. In a small trial, lozenges shortened colds when taken in the first 24 hours after symptoms developed.

The bottom line? Vitamin C and zinc won't prevent a cold, but they may shorten the cold you already have. Check with your doctor before starting supplements.

Eat nutrient-dense foods to prevent deficiency. If you're low in vitamin C or zinc, you're more susceptible to illness, so it's a good idea to work these nutrients into your regular diet.

Did you know you can eat 94% of your daily vitamin C recommendation in one large kiwi? Just 3 ounces of oysters affords you 674% of your daily zinc. Grains, baked beans, chickpeas, and nuts are also good sources of zinc.

Colon cancer

3 flavorful ways to fight inflammation's fire

Bang. You stubbed your toe, and now it's starting to swell and turn red. You're probably familiar with this kind of inflammation — white blood cells rushing toward the affected area for protection. But inflammation doesn't just come from trauma. It can come from your diet, too.

A Western diet with lots of meat and refined grains is more inflammatory than a Mediterranean diet, one filled with legumes, fatty fish, and fruits and vegetables. And since inflammation, especially chronic, can increase your risk of colon cancer, so can a Western diet.

Cancer of the colon or rectum is also called colorectal cancer. Although it is the fourth most common cancer in the United States, colorectal cancer is often curable if you catch it early enough.

Symptoms can include blood in the stool, narrower stools, a change in bowel habits, and general stomach discomfort. However, you may not develop symptoms right away, so screening is important. Everyone who is 50 or older should be screened regularly.

Eating the right foods and nutrients may also help you avoid this devastating disease. And you don't have to sacrifice flavor for health. Spice up your dishes with these fantastic anti-inflammatories.

Alliums are super inflammation-fighters. If you're the type of person who loves to pile on the

Eat

Cabbage	Broccoli
Jicama	Chia seeds
Legumes	Turmeric
Hops	Ginger
Onions	Garlic
Yogurt	Potatoes
Wheat bran	Rice bran

Avoid

Processed meat
Red meat

onions and garlic, you're doing your colon a big favor. Research has shown these vegetables — members of the allium family — have anti-inflammatory powers.

In a large Chinese study of over 800 people, researchers found that eating allium vegetables was associated with a lower colon cancer risk for both men and women.

Onions get an extra boost from fisetin, a super flavonoid with exceptional anti-inflammatory powers. In a recent small study, people undergoing chemotherapy received either 100 milligrams of fisetin or a placebo each day for seven weeks. At the end of that time, two blood markers of inflammation were significantly reduced in the fisetin group.

A spice that kills cancer cells better than chemotherapy drugs? Surprising but true. Not only does ginger do a number on colon cancer, in one lab study it killed ovarian cancer cells as well as or better than chemo drugs. Ginger provides a one-two punch by prompting some cells to commit suicide and others to self-digest.

Because inflammation plays such a big role in the spread of cancer, scientists think fisetin could be helpful as an "antitumor agent."

Ginger gets your body's defenses going. Pour yourself a cup of ginger tea, or add some fresh ginger to your favorite stir-fry, and you'll help reduce your risk of colon cancer. Ginger is well-known for its antioxidant and anti-inflammation properties.

Numerous lab and animal studies have shown that ginger and its active compounds keep colorectal cancer cells from growing and spreading. And ginger is a team player. Studies have found it helps strengthen the anti-cancer effects of some chemotherapy drugs.

Turmeric takes out colon cancer. If you're a fan of turmeric, you have curcumin to thank for its beautiful orange color and many of its health benefits. Curcumin is anti-inflammatory, and animal and lab studies suggest it may help prevent colon cancer.

COX-2, a catalyst that speeds up chemical reactions, is particularly known for promoting cancer. Studies have found that targeting COX-2 with nonsteroidal anti-inflammatory drugs (NSAIDs) can reduce colon cancer risk. And experts have observed that curcumin works like NSAIDs to block COX-2, so it may also help protect your colon.

You can reap the benefits of curcumin by sprinkling turmeric on a variety of dishes. But talk to your doctor first before adding large amounts to your diet.

The No. 1 thing you need to keep your colon healthy

Think you get enough fiber? Think again. As many as 95 in 100 Americans don't meet their daily recommended intake.

Compared to those who eat the least dietary fiber, observational data suggests that those who eat the most have a 15% to 30% decrease in colorectal cancer as well as heart disease, stroke, and diabetes. Even if you've already been diagnosed with colon cancer, dietary fiber may reduce your fatality risk.

Experts think fiber helps fight cancer by increasing stool bulk and decreasing the amount of time it spends in your colon. It may also dilute cancer-causing agents in your gastrointestinal tract. Try these three great sources to fill up your fiber tank.

Ch-ch-ch-chia seeds give you the fiber you need. Chia seeds may be tiny, but they're a powerful way to clean out your digestive tract, which reduces your risk for diseases like colon cancer. Just 1 tablespoon of chia seeds provides

High levels of magnesium in your diet are associated with a lower risk of colon cancer. But many Americans don't get enough of this important mineral through their meals. Add foods like rice and wheat bran to your dish rotation for a magnesium boost.

4 grams (g) of insoluble fiber. The recommended daily fiber intake for adults over age 50 is 21 g for women and 30 g for men.

You may have noticed these seeds come in different colors. There's no nutritional difference between the black and white seeds, but brown ones aren't fully matured.

Eat them raw by adding them to a salad or smoothie or baking them into foods like crackers and bread. Just be sure you mix them with something. The seeds make a gel when they touch liquids, and that can make them hard to swallow if eaten alone.

Beans are the fiber source you know and love to spice up. They're diverse in size and color, but their names can be misleading. Navy beans are actually white, but luckily, their nutrition is straightforward.

Beans provide a lot of fiber, which alone can help fend off colon cancer. But their benefits don't stop there. One study following colon cancer survivors found that navy beans increased the bacterial richness of the subjects' gut microbiome. Colon cancer risk is associated with lower numbers of good bacteria, so you can protect yourself by adding these powerhouses to your diet.

If you find beans bland, consider boosting their flavor with one of the foods in the story *3 flavorful ways to fight inflammation's fire*.

Bran brings cancer protection — and bonuses. Bran has the brawn to fight cancer. Its combo of fiber and phytochemicals makes it a fierce ally in your gut.

- In a small study of colon cancer survivors, researchers found that eating rice bran for one month increased certain metabolites in plasma and urine that protect against cancer. Another study showed that eating brown rice, which contains the bran, just once a week cut polyp risk by 40%. Rice bran also adds to the richness and diversity of the gut microbiome, which is important for a healthy colon.

- Prefer wheat bran? Try a breakfast like Kellogg's Bran Flakes, a rich source of natural grain fiber. Eating this kind of cereal daily can help prevent constipation and weight gain in addition to colon cancer. That's because eating lots of fiber is associated with lower body weight. And common causes of constipation include a low-fiber diet and not drinking enough fluids. So fill your plate with fiber-packed fruits and veggies alongside your bran to get your body in tiptop shape.

This veggie is your ace against cancer

What's cheap, low-calorie, and green all over? Cabbage. And when it comes to major ailments, cabbage is a jack-of-all-trades. It's a proven cancer crusher and may also help against clogged arteries, obesity, and diabetes. Here's why you should add cabbage to your dinner plate tonight.

Foolproof fiber content fights cancer. Cabbage is a cruciferous vegetable. It's part of a family of fiber-packed veggies that also includes broccoli, cauliflower, kale, radishes, and watercress. Cabbage's power against colon cancer comes in part from its crunch punch of fiber.

Experts say the fiber could be working in several ways. One is that it helps move food through your digestive tract more quickly, which reduces the chances of problems developing.

Healthy compounds offer superstar protection. Cabbage's benefits are not limited to its fiber. Cruciferous vegetables like cabbage contain glucosinolates, compounds that give these foods their bitter taste. And research has found they're superstars when it comes to fighting cancer.

Here's why. When glucosinolates break down, they form isothiocyanates (ITCs). Two major ITCs are benzyl isothiocyanate (BITC) and sulforaphane (SFN), and they're both found in cabbage.

- BITC encourages colon cancer cells to commit suicide and also blocks tumor cells from spreading.

- SFN plays a role in stopping colon cancer growth by damaging the DNA of cancer cells.

Thanks to these compounds, eating cabbage is associated with a reduced risk of colon cancer. Studies confirm it's also effective on breast, bladder, brain, lung, and stomach cancer.

Preparation is key to a colon cancer shutdown. To get the full benefits of cruciferous veggies, it's best to eat them raw. Chewing or chopping them will convert the glucosinolate into ITCs. Cooking them results in fewer of these cancer fighters for your body to absorb. Light cooking, like steaming for less than five minutes, will save some of the ITCs.

Luckily, raw cabbage is a delicious addition to salads and slaws. If you turn it into sauerkraut, you'll get an additional health boost from the probiotics that develop in fermented foods.

Discover jicama and the easy way to eat this fiber-filled food

If you imagine an onion-shaped potato, you'll end up picturing jicama, pronounced HEE-kah-ma or HIK-ah-ma. Native to Mexico, this root vegetable is mild, slightly sweet, and rich with fiber — almost 7 grams in 1 cup. That's about a quarter of your daily requirement.

To take advantage of this nutritious veggie, here's a hint for preparation. When it comes to taking off the skin, skip the peeler. Instead, tackle the tough outer layer with a chef's knife.

First cut off the root's top and bottom to create two flat surfaces. Then, laying the jicama on its longest flat side, slice under the skin moving top to bottom to remove all of it. Then slice and dice as you please.

Jicama is often eaten raw, so keep it simple and serve it on a salad or as a crudité. Or add it to your recipes for salsa, spring rolls, or slaw.

Make room for legumes — your colon cancer kicker

Say "soy you later, alligator" to red and processed meat if you want to avoid colon cancer. Legumes should be your first choice for protein, experts say.

Researchers looked at dietary patterns and disease risk as part of the Adventist Health Study. They found that people who ate legumes more than two times a week were nearly 50% less likely to develop colon cancer, compared to those who ate them less than once a week or none at all.

And new research continues to support the benefits of legumes, a class of vegetables that includes beans, peas, and lentils. For example, Chinese scientists investigated data from 14 studies with more than a million participants and concluded that eating more legumes was associated with a decreased risk of colorectal cancer.

The fiber in legumes may be one reason they're so successful at fighting cancer. But their greatest health powers may lie with their phytoestrogens. Two common dietary phytoestrogens — isoflavones and lignans — are both found in legumes and may have cancer-fighting properties.

Soybeans are an especially rich source of isoflavones, which have a structure similar to estrogen. They can bind with estrogen receptors, crowding out natural estrogen, which reduces your cancer risk.

Studies have found that too much estrogen in your body puts you at higher risk for some cancers, including colon cancer. Isoflavones may also stop the growth of cancer cells.

Eastern populations with diets rich in soy foods have traditionally seen low rates of colorectal cancer, scientists say. By adding soybeans and other legumes to your diet, you can follow in their footsteps.

Don't worry, be hoppy: The surprising ingredient that can help you fight cancer

You may be familiar with hops as a key ingredient in beer. It gives it its flavor and color. Now scientists have found hops may do something else — battle cancer, including colon cancer.

The common hop plant produces the flavonoid xanthohumol (XN), pronounced zan-thoh-hugh-moll. Studies following the anti-cancer effects of XN have found it can kill cancer cells and suppress tumor development.

The good news is you don't have to drink beer to reap the benefit of hops. Spent hops, what's left after brewing beer, can be used in bread or baked into nutritious energy bars. Your local brewery may be happy to supply you with some.

You can also add fresh hops petals to stew, or sprinkle them on pasta or bruschetta. Use them sparingly though — they have a strong bitter flavor.

Look for hops online at *walmart.com* and *amazon.com* or specialty stores like *freshops.com*. If you want an unusual addition to your herb garden, try growing them yourself.

Men: Scoop up the benefits of yogurt

Yogurt is a perfect snack, smoothie ingredient, and more. That's great because the more you eat it, the more your colon may benefit.

A recent study found that men who ate at least two servings of yogurt per week had a lower risk of developing polyps than those who never ate yogurt. These abnormal tissue growths in your colon may or may not become cancerous.

The study pulled information from almost three decades of data that included more than 32,000 men and 55,000 women. Researchers found that the men's risk for ordinary polyps was

19% lower when they ate yogurt twice a week. Their risk was 26% lower for precancerous growths. However, no association between yogurt and polyp risk was found in women.

Although this doesn't mean yogurt prevented the polyp growth, experts say yogurt probiotics like *Lactobacillus bulgaricus* and *Streptococcus thermophilus* may help reduce cancer causers like inflammation.

Another nutrient in yogurt that may boost its healthful potential? Vitamin D. Many yogurts are fortified with the sunshine vitamin, and having more than enough vitamin D in your body is associated with a lower risk of colon cancer.

So if you're adding yogurt to your diet, keep it low fat or fat free, and look for brands with both probiotics and vitamin D to help keep your colon healthy.

Rice and potatoes — they're better for you than you think

Rice, pasta, and potatoes may be superheroes in the fight against colon cancer, thanks to a type of starch your body can't digest, dubbed "resistant starch."

Acting like fiber, resistant starch makes its way from your mouth to your colon without undergoing much change. While in your colon, it ferments and becomes a prebiotic, feeding the good bacteria in your bowels. That good bacteria creates a fatty acid called butyrate that lowers the pH level in your colon, pares down inflammation, and stops cancer cells from growing.

This special starch occurs naturally in certain foods like green, unripe bananas as well as seeds, grains, and legumes. You also create it when you cook, then cool, starchy foods. So keep eating your favorite cold pasta, rice, and potato salads — your colon is reaping the benefit.

Depression

Grapes pick you up when you're feeling down

If you've ever wondered why you feel more relaxed after drinking red wine, it may be because of resveratrol in the grapes. Studies show this polyphenol can help decrease symptoms of depression.

But before you grab a glass, remember that its other ingredient — alcohol — can worsen them. And if you take antidepressants, the mix may be dangerous. Your best bet? Stick to grapes and berries instead.

How to tell if depression is wearing you down. Depression is caused by chemical changes in your body. Specifically, imbalances in the neurotransmitters serotonin, norepinephrine, and dopamine that control your mood. These chemicals act as messengers within your brain, so an imbalance can send the wrong message.

Clinical depression is a serious disease that calls for serious help from an expert. But how can you tell if your blue mood is true depression? It may be the difference between needing a push to go out with friends and refusing to go out at all, or wanting to change certain things about your life compared to feeling trapped in your life.

Keep in mind that depression may show up differently depending on your age. Older people don't always feel sad or worthless when they're depressed. They might be tired and grumpy instead. In fact, some of the signs of depression in the elderly — memory loss, restlessness, and confusion — are often misdiagnosed as dementia.

Eat

Grapes	Berries
Dark chocolate	Bananas
Nuts	Greens
Black-eyed peas	Turkey
Butternut squash	Tea

Avoid

Ultra-processed foods like chips, soft drinks, and sweet cereals

Fend off depression with resveratrol's three-pronged attack.
Researchers have found in animal studies that resveratrol helps
fight depression. In one study, it
worked as well as the antidepressants fluoxetine, desipramine,
and ketamine. Plus it has
limited side effects, unlike
common antidepressants such
as selective serotonin reuptake
inhibitors (SSRIs). That could
make it a great alternative or
addition to current treatments.

> Depression can suck you of
> your appetite and energy, but
> you'll only feel worse if you
> don't eat. Fill up with a green
> smoothie — no cooking
> required. Leafy greens like
> spinach are dense with anti-
> depressant nutrients. Balance
> every 2 cups of greens with 3
> cups of fruit and 2 cups of
> liquid for the best flavor.

Here's how experts think resveratrol works against depression.

- Resveratrol plays a role in the hypothalamic-pituitary-adrenal
  (HPA) axis. The HPA axis is your "stress circuit" — it controls
  the hormones that respond to stress. Cortisol is your main
  stress hormone, and it rises when you're depressed. But
  resveratrol can lower your levels and regulate the HPA axis.

- People with depression often have more inflammation, and
  resveratrol has an anti-inflammatory effect. That's especially
  helpful because inflammation can stop neurogenesis — your
  body's process of making your brain and nervous system's
  building blocks, called neurons. Neurotransmitters like serotonin
  carry messages between neurons and other parts of the body.

- Brain-derived neurotrophic factor (BDNF) is a protein that
  plays a role in proper brain health. One of its jobs is to build
  and maintain the brain circuits that neurotransmitters travel
  on. Chronic stress can lower BDNF levels, but in animal
  studies, resveratrol increased them.

Even though scientists need more information about resveratrol's
effects in people, they're encouraged by their positive results so
far. If you're feeling blue, try adding more red and purple grapes
and berries to your diet to see if they help lift your mood.

Fight depression with the right foods

Eating healthier is a surefire way to fight off depression symptoms like tiredness and trouble concentrating. Studies have shown that changing your diet can have a greater impact on depression than a social support group. But if you're not sure where to start, these two diets make your job simple. Follow their guidelines to boost the benefits of your food choices.

Win the 100-meter DASH against depression. The Dietary Approaches to Stop Hypertension (DASH) diet recommends fat-free or low-fat dairy products, fruits, and vegetables. And it limits foods high in sugar and saturated fats.

The diet was developed to help improve blood pressure, but studies have found it can help with other conditions such as depression. A recent study of 964 elderly people found that those who closely followed the DASH diet were 11% less likely to develop depression than those who strayed furthest from it.

Other health problems like stroke and heart disease are common in people with depression. So even though researchers aren't sure if the DASH diet directly impacts depression levels, they know that eating a healthy diet with more fruits and vegetables can improve your blood pressure and other health difficulties. And that can make you feel better all around.

Live like you're on the Mediterranean. It looks like fresh fruits, vegetables, and whole grains benefit more than just your physical health. New research says following a Mediterranean-style diet may be the key to ridding yourself of depression.

That's according to Australian scientists who recruited 67 depressed adults for a three-month study. Each ate a relatively unhealthy diet that was heavy on sweets, salty snacks, and processed meats like hot dogs and salami. Most were being treated for their depression.

Once the study began, half the participants adopted a Mediterranean-style diet rich in vegetables, fruits, whole grains, and olive oil. The other half kept their old eating habits. Guess what happened after 12 weeks? More than 30% of the people on the Mediterranean-style diet were no longer depressed. That compares with 8% in the other group.

The researchers didn't give a reason for the results. But a previous Spanish study on depression and the Mediterranean diet says those foods may fight inflammation, improve blood flow, and repair cell damage. That, in turn, could lower your risk of becoming depressed.

Go bananas for this healthy, mood-lifting treat

Sometimes a little goodie will give you a pick-me-up when you're feeling down. Choose one filled with blues-busting magnesium, and you'll give your mind and body an extra boost.

Studies show that increasing the magnesium in your diet can decrease depression symptoms in mild to moderate cases. And from top to bottom, chocolate-covered bananas have the power of magnesium on their side. Plus they're easy to make.

Dip your banana in melted dark chocolate to supercharge it. Chocolate is packed with even more magnesium than bananas. Dark chocolate especially may reduce the symptoms of depression, so pick a bar with at least 70% cocoa.

While the chocolate is still wet, sprinkle on crushed nuts. Almonds and peanuts will both add an extra boost of magnesium. Then freeze it until the chocolate is solid, and get ready for a sweet, feel-good treat.

Put a lid on depression the Mediterranean way

Want to create your own mood-boosting meals? Here's what participants ate during the three-month study on the Mediterranean diet and depression.

Food	Servings
whole grains	5-8 daily
vegetables	6 daily
fruit	3 daily
legumes	3-4 weekly
low-fat, unsweetened dairy	2 daily
raw, unsalted nuts	1 daily
fish	at least 2 weekly
lean red meat	3-4 weekly
chicken	2-3 weekly
eggs	up to 6 weekly

Don't forget to include 3 tablespoons of olive oil in your diet each day. Limit red wine to two glasses a day at mealtime. And have no more than three servings a week of "extras" such as sweets, fried foods, processed meats, and refined cereal.

These soup-er meals take a bite out of depression

When the cold months roll around each year, the time change may make you feel like you're falling back into moods as dark as the newly unlit sky. If your depression seems to cycle with the seasons, you may have seasonal affective disorder (SAD).

This negative mood change most commonly starts in late fall or early winter and melts away with the return of sunnier days in spring and summer.

SAD may drain you of energy or even change your appetite. But the best cold weather food, soup, may be the perfect remedy. It warms you up inside and gives you the nutrients you need to fend off depression. Whether you have SAD or just feel sad, these comfort soups can help bring your spirits up.

Before your mood goes south, try this soul food specialty. Black-eyed pea soup is a staple in the southern states, and it can hit the spot on a cold day, while the folate in it can help lift your mood. Low levels of folate are associated with depression. Around 1 in 3 people being treated for the condition have a folate deficiency.

Studies have established that folate has a positive effect against depression in animals, and they suggest people may also benefit. Scientists think folate helps produce S-adenosylmethionine (SAM) which affects neurotransmitters like serotonin and dopamine that play a role in mood and depression.

Gobble up turkey noodle soup to relax and rejuvenate. Turkey is often blamed for making you feel sleepy after eating, but that may not be true. What scientists do know is that tryptophan, which is in turkey, helps ward off depression.

Would you believe your gut can play a big part in how you feel? Stress can cause changes in your microbiome, and these changes can then impact your mood. Researchers think tryptophan is involved in this series of events.

Your body changes tryptophan into serotonin, and studies have found that increasing its levels in your digestive system has a positive effect on your brain. That means if you focus on your microbiome and what you eat, you may help yourself feel better.

Enjoy the soothing creaminess of butternut squash. Add some color to your plate with butternut squash soup. It's chock-full of antidepressant nutrients like the antioxidant beta carotene, which gives it its brilliant orange color.

Scientists have found a connection between beta carotene and depression that suggests the less beta carotene a person has, the more likely they are to be depressed.

That may be because this potent antioxidant protects the brain from oxidative stress that can damage and reduce the number of neurotransmitters you have. And having fewer neurotransmitters is associated with depression.

Avoid these foods that drag you down

When you're feeling blue, it's easy to reach for a bag of chips or a pint of ice cream, hoping to make yourself feel better. But let's face it, they usually make you feel worse. And it's not just from guilt.

Scientists have found that having ultra-processed food (UPF) in your diet is associated with a greater risk of depression. A study with data from over 25,000 people found more cases of depression in groups who ate more UPF.

These foods have been processed so many times they've lost almost all their essential nutrients and fiber. Plus they're often high in sugar and additives. Think of soft drinks, sweet cereals, and other packaged foods.

Focusing on fresh produce and minimally processed foods like grains and legumes is your best option. If you do eat packaged foods, look for those with few changes or additions, like canned beans and tuna.

The healing power of tea time

The soothing rhythm of preparing tea may do wonders for your mental state. But the biggest benefit may be in the tea itself. Drinking 1 or more cups a day is an easy way to get nutrients that work together to fight depression.

Researchers believe the combination of chemicals in tea, rather than one in particular, may give tea its anti-depression powers. Each makes a small change that leads to an overall difference in your mood.

Multifunctional tea takes down depression. Like grapes, tea impacts the major paths scientists believe control depression. For instance, your HPA axis manages your fight-or-flight response. If stress causes it to operate continuously, referred to as HPA axis hyperactivity, it can overwhelm you and lead to symptoms of depression. But the polyphenols in tea may help normalize its activity.

Tea has also been shown to lower inflammation, help rebalance neurotransmitters like serotonin and dopamine, and fight oxidation that damages neurons — all of which can lead to depression.

Keep the cups flowing for best results. Don't worry about what kind of tea you're drinking for now. Scientists aren't sure which type is the best, and since each tea has its own beneficial qualities, your best bet may actually be to drink multiple types regularly.

What matters more is how much you drink. Studies have found that a higher consumption of tea is linked with lower risk of depression.

- In an analysis of 11 studies, researchers found that for every 3 cups of tea you drink in a day there is an associated 37% decrease in risk of depression.

- Examination of a Korean survey of health and nutrition found that those who drank more than 3 cups of green tea in a week had 21% lower rates of depression.

Aging populations especially seem to benefit from tea's depression-reducing effects. However, it works best in mild to moderate cases and may not make a significant dent in severe depression.

Diabetes

Take a deep dive to sink your blood sugar

Don't let the dreaded D word haunt your retirement years. Diabetes affects almost 1 out of every 10 Americans. The most common form of this disease — known as type 2 diabetes — develops when your body can't produce enough insulin to keep your blood sugar in check. And your risk of getting diabetes increases as you age, or if you're overweight.

Over time, this can cause heart disease, nerve damage, and kidney problems. Fortunately, you can lower your risk just by eating the right foods. The first place you should look? Under the sea.

Feast on fish to fight back against diabetes. Most people don't add fat to their diets when they want to be healthier. But the right fats can crush your risk of diabetes.

In a small study, Norwegian researchers discovered fatty fish like salmon, mackerel, or sardines can help control your blood sugar. Scientists asked a group of overweight adults to eat about a pound and a half of fish every week.

At the end of the eight-week study, the results showed that eating fish rich in omega-3 helped keep post-meal blood sugar spikes at bay.

Already have diabetes? Don't skimp on the fish. A trial published in *JAMA Ophthalmology* found that eating 500 grams of omega-3s a week can cut your risk of diabetic retinopathy by 46%. You'll get almost three times that in a 3 3/4-ounce can of sardines.

Eat

Fatty fish	Seaweed
Cabbage	Jicama
Milk	Blueberries
Peaches	Guava
Pecans	Cinnamon
Low-fat yogurt	Oats

Avoid

Soda
Fruit juice
White potatoes
White bread and pasta

Tame your blood sugar with a bit of "kelp" from this surprising source. The sea holds more diabetes protection than you might think. Recently, Japanese researchers found that people who eat a lot of seaweed, soy, and mushrooms are less likely to need medications for diabetes.

Scientists think the credit goes to the fiber, antioxidants, and other nutrients in these three foods.

And on the other side of the globe, Norwegian researchers discovered seaweed is powerful even when eaten alone. An animal study revealed that these aquatic plants improve insulin sensitivity by slowing the breakdown and digestion of sugars.

Exactly how much seaweed you should eat daily isn't quite clear. But if you don't usually eat plants from the sea, why not give them a try? You can find dried seaweed online, in Asian markets, and sometimes in the international section of your local grocery store.

New to seaweed?
Here's what you need to know

You can enjoy seaweed on your dinner plate even if you live thousands of miles away from the ocean. All you need to know is where to look.

Dried seaweed can often be found at Asian marts or ordered online. And it's all sold under different names. For example, depending on the variety, seaweed could be sold as nori, dulse, wakame, or arame. Experts recommend steering clear of any seaweed sold under the name Hijiki, because it often contains high levels of arsenic.

You can eat the dried sheets of seaweed by themselves, or blitz it in a blender and sprinkle it onto food instead of adding salt.

If you're not a big fan of the flavor on its own, put some into your soup a few minutes before you're ready to eat. The flavor will mellow as the seaweed softens.

Crunch on cabbage to win your battle with diabetes

Steamed, baked, raw, or even fermented — no matter how you cook your cabbage, this tasty treat could hold the key to staving off diabetes. That's because it's loaded with vitamin K, which is one of the most important nutrients you can get. But not all vitamin K is the same. Here's what you need to know.

Crush your risk when you call on vitamin K1. In a recent study published in *Diabetes*, researchers examined data from three previous studies that included hundreds of thousands of participants. And they found that those who showed the highest levels of vitamin K1 — also known as phylloquinone — were least likely to develop type 2 diabetes.

The exact cause isn't known, but the leading theory points to vitamin K1's role in creating osteocalcin. This protein, which also helps build up your skeleton, is an important part of insulin production. If you run low on osteocalcin, you're at greater risk of developing insulin resistance.

So how can you get more vitamin K1? Cabbage and other leafy green vegetables are your best bet. Men should get 120 micrograms (mcg) every day, while women need 90 mcg. You can get 67 mcg in a single cup of chopped, raw cabbage.

Protect your pancreas with fermented foods. Phylloquinone isn't the only K vitamin you should add to your diet. Researchers from China believe its cousin — vitamin K2 or menaquinone — may be even more powerful at preventing diabetes. In a review of multiple studies, they found evidence that suggests for every 10 mcg of vitamin K2 you eat, you reduce your risk of diabetes by 7%.

Vitamin K2 may be stronger simply because it's easier for your body to absorb and use this nutrient. So where do you find this half of the vitamin K duo? Your digestive system converts some of the K1 you eat into K2, but, unfortunately, it's not an efficient process.

Fermented foods are a great source of vitamin K2. So the next time you pick up some cabbage, consider turning it into a tangy sauerkraut. You'll also find K2 in egg yolks, hard cheeses, and organ meats like liver.

Root out blood sugar spikes with this exotic veggie

If you have diabetes, you probably know that potatoes are practically verboten. Their high glycemic index means these starchy tubers are guaranteed to cause a blood sugar spike.

But if you miss eating them, there's another food you might want to try. Jicama — also known as the Mexican potato — is a great alternative. An animal study found this root vegetable could help boost your insulin sensitivity and lower your blood sugar.

Jicama has a low glycemic index, so you can munch away without worrying about your next glucose test. Plus it's loaded with fiber like inulin, a prebiotic that feeds the good bacteria in your gut. Fiber also makes you feel full longer, which helps with weight loss — another good way to fight diabetes.

Say nuts to diabetes with these mighty minerals

Worried about bringing down your blood sugar? Fortunately, it can be as easy as eating one food — nuts.

In a recent small study in *Nutrients*, researchers from Tufts University fed overweight volunteers a control diet with no nuts for four weeks. Then they asked those people to add a small handful of pecans to their meals. After another four weeks, the volunteers improved their insulin resistance, lowered their cholesterol, and brought down their triglycerides.

"Pecans are naturally high in monounsaturated and polyunsaturated fats, so replacing a portion of the saturated fat in the diet with these healthier fats can explain some of the cardioprotective effects we observed," says lead researcher Diane McKay, Ph.D.

"But pecans also contain a number of bioactive plant compounds as well as vitamins and essential minerals that all likely contributed to this benefit," she says. In fact, most nuts are great sources of two minerals that are proven to help you fend off diabetes.

Call on zinc to shore up your blood sugar. A handful of nuts can get you over 12% of your daily recommendation for zinc. And that's great news if you're battling diabetes.

The data shows that the more zinc you have in your body, the better you can prevent or manage diabetes. A recent meta-analysis of 32 studies revealed that supplementing with this powerful mineral can reduce blood sugar concentrations and inflammation and increase your sensitivity to insulin.

Experts say men should aim for 11 milligrams (mg) of zinc a day, and women should get 8 mg. You can get more zinc in other nuts, plus it's in foods like pumpkin seeds, shellfish, and meat.

Need a little help managing diabetes? Manganese can make it easy. Another reason scientists think nuts might help you win the war on diabetes is due to their high manganese content. A single ounce of pecans has over half of your daily needs.

This nutrient plays a role in helping your body digest and absorb sugar. A number of animal studies suggest manganese can help improve glucose tolerance, but the research is still out on humans. In the meantime, women should aim to get 1.8 mg of manganese daily, while men need about 2.3 mg.

But be careful not to overdo it. One study suggested that getting too much of this mineral could increase your risk of diabetes, too.

3 fabulous fruits that fight diabetes

You've heard of Huey, Dewey, and Louie. And you definitely know about snap, crackle, and pop. But what about peaches, blueberries, and guava? The last trio may not be as famous, but this trifecta is one you'll want to know more about — especially if you have diabetes.

Pick peaches to blunt your blood sugar. In a recent study, Chinese researchers found that peaches could be one of the best fruits you can eat to fight diabetes. You might not think these sweet treats could offer potent protection, but they're chock-full of polyphenols that can help you manage your blood sugar. And one in particular — called myricetin — may hold the key to winning the war on diabetes.

Scientists examined the diets of over 24,000 people. They found that those who ate the most myricetin-rich foods — like peaches, apples, and oranges — were least likely to have type 2 diabetes. The researchers think this polyphenol's strong antioxidant activity may have a protective effect against the disease.

Snack on blueberries to help your body use insulin. Want to fend off those dreaded glucose spikes? Sprinkle a few blueberries into your next salad. These powerful little berries are loaded with chemicals known as anthocyanins. They give these fruits their distinctive, dark blue color. And more importantly, experts think these compounds can prompt your body to release insulin into your blood.

In a study published by the *Journal of Nutrition*, researchers split senior adults with diabetes into two groups. Half of them took a placebo, while the others took anthocyanin supplements designed to mimic the effects of eating a serving of blueberries.

After 24 weeks, the people who took the anthocyanin supplements

These three fruits are not just great diabetes fighters. They could help you fend off obesity, too. That's because peaches, guava, and blueberries are chock-full of fiber, which helps you eat less and still feel full.

improved their insulin sensitivity. That means the cells of their bodies were better at using insulin, which helps lower their blood sugar.

Call on guava to keep sugar in check. If guava isn't on your grocery list, it needs to be. Scientists say this South American superfruit will help you blunt high blood sugar.

A study recently published in *Nutrients* revealed that this food can help block your gut from absorbing too much sugar. Austrian researchers asked one group of volunteers to drink a sugary solution with guava added to it, while another group only had sugar in their drinks.

After two hours, the scientists took blood samples and examined them. Surprisingly, the guava group had significantly lower blood sugar. The experts aren't sure exactly why guava is so powerful, but they think the credit lies with the variety of polyphenols found in this fruit.

Got milk? 2 ways dairy helps you fend off high blood sugar

Can you drink milk? If so, you're a rare bird. Only 1 in 3 adults worldwide can properly digest the sugar — called lactose — in milk. But this might be a lifesaver if you're at risk for diabetes. That's because experts say the more dairy you eat and drink, the less likely you are to get type 2 diabetes.

This fantastic vitamin puts the "d" in dairy. Experts think one of the biggest reasons milk and other dairy products can help you win the battle against diabetes is because they're loaded with vitamin D.

To get an idea of just how powerful this nutrient is, take a look at a recent study published by researchers from Université Laval in Quebec. Scientists divided up 96 adults with type 2 diabetes or prediabetes. Half of them took a placebo pill, while the others took a high-dose vitamin D supplement. After six months, the supplement group improved their insulin resistance.

People in the study took 125 micrograms of vitamin D daily. To get that through diet alone, you'd have to drink around 50 cups of milk every day. So this might be a good time to consider a supplement. Just be sure to get your doctor's approval before taking any high-dose vitamins.

Taurine in dairy will amp up your insulin. Researchers noticed that people with type 2 diabetes often run low on taurine. And that's bad news. This essential amino acid helps keep your blood sugar stable by telling your pancreas to release more insulin into your bloodstream.

Experts think not having enough taurine in your body may play a part in your developing the disease. And if you have diabetes, make sure you're getting enough. Research has shown this nutrient can help fight complications, like nerve and kidney damage.

So how much do you need every day? Your best bet is to include plenty of taurine-rich foods in your diet like milk, cheese, and shellfish.

Stop diabetes from getting on your nerves with ALC

Symptoms can be so subtle you barely notice them — just a slight tingling in your feet. Then may come shooting pain at night, by patches of numbness up to your ankles. Within months you can be so unsteady on your feet that you fear falling and breaking a bone.

The diagnosis? Peripheral neuropathy — a condition affecting up to half of all people with diabetes. The cause? Chronically high blood sugar levels that damage the nerves in their feet. Fortunately, many people find relief through medication, a healthy diet, and exercise — all of which help keep blood sugar levels in check.

New research suggests that taking supplements of the amino acid acetyl-L-carnitine (ALC) may lessen the pain associated with diabetic neuropathy and improve nerve function. Why? ALC may provide the extra energy nerve cells need to regenerate while also helping your brain produce natural painkillers.

For folks who want to try out acetyl-L-carnitine supplements, experts at the Linus Pauling Institute recommend a daily dose of 500 to 1,000 milligrams. But before you start taking ALC, be sure to check with your doctor, particularly if you take beta blockers, blood thinners, or thyroid medication.

Call on this humble spice to lower your blood sugar

Would you believe that cinnamon oils can help heal wounds? Even better, studies have shown this spice can lower your cholesterol and blood pressure, fight inflammation and cancer, and fend off fatigue and food poisoning. It's even on the cutting edge of Alzheimer's prevention.

But the best part? Sprinkling a bit more of this sweet spice on your meals may help you fight back against diabetes.

In a recent meta-analysis, researchers examined multiple studies and found cinnamon can lower your fasting blood sugar and even improve your insulin resistance. But other research findings have been mixed.

If you want to give it a try, talk to your doctor about a safe amount to take. Some studies have used up to 6 grams of cinnamon a day, which is about 2 1/3 teaspoons. If you have liver problems, eating too much cinnamon could make them worse. So be smart and take your doctor's advice.

Keep your sugar on track with a little help from your gut

Have you heard of the microbiome? It's the term scientists use for the trillions of bacteria that live in your gut. Experts think this ecosystem inside of you could hold the key to fighting off everything from Alzheimer's to cancer. And now researchers even think the answer to fighting off diabetes is there, too.

Enjoy the power of probiotics. Think of your gut like a garden. All the care and attention you give to your plants just can't seem to hold off a horde of aphids. The solution? Bring in a few ladybugs. They'll keep those bad bugs from gnawing on your tomatoes.

Probiotics can do the same thing for you. Scientists say the helpful bacteria that swarm your microbiome may be a new way to control type 2 diabetes.

In a recent meta-analysis of 12 studies, experts found that adding *lactobacilli* and *bifidobacteria* to your diet could help fight blood sugar spikes and insulin resistance.

These strains of bacteria are easy to find in probiotic supplements, yogurts, and drinks. Just make sure to look for products with live cultures that aren't out of date.

Feast on fiber to amp up your microbiome. In a Chinese study, researchers assigned people with type 2 diabetes into one of two groups. Participants in both groups followed standard diet recommendations for their condition and took a prescription drug to control their blood sugar. But only one group ate a large variety of fiber with their diet.

After 12 weeks, the fiber-eaters improved their A1C levels — their average blood sugar over three months — and lowered their fasting glucose levels. An added benefit? They lost weight.

Experts think this high-fiber diet was so effective because it was loaded with prebiotics — nutrients that feed the beneficial bacteria in your gut. In turn, these bacteria help your body produce more insulin and control your blood sugar.

To reap the same benefits, load up on foods rich in fiber like oats, barley, and beans.

Fatigue

Sideline sluggishness with these supermarket solutions

Tired of feeling tired? Your diet may be to blame. After all, food has a big impact on your energy level. Think of your body as a high-performance engine. Feed it low-octane fuel — lots of fried foods, sugary drinks, and salty snacks, for example — and you're bound to see decreased power and performance.

Want to make sure you're firing on all cylinders? Jump-starting your diet could put these fatigue-causing conditions to rest.

Watermelon keeps dehydration at bay. It turns out that even a mild case of dehydration can wear you out. That's according to a study of young women who were given mental tests while slightly dehydrated and, on a later occasion, while fully hydrated. The women reported being less able to concentrate and more fatigued after a loss of just 1.36% of their bodies' normal water volume.

The results support what scientists already know — without enough water, your body simply can't function normally.

Snack on these water-rich foods to keep hydrated.

- watermelon, strawberries, and cantaloupe

- cucumber, lettuce, and celery

- yogurt, cottage cheese, and fat-free milk

Eat

Watermelon	Lentils
Brussels sprouts	Mackerel
Dark chocolate	Oysters
Chicken liver	Eggs

Avoid

High-glycemic foods like instant mashed potatoes, white bread, and white rice

Heavily processed foods like deli meat, sweetened cereal, and frozen pizza

Fatty fish keeps cells well fed. Ever hear of adenosine triphosphate? Dubbed ATP for short, it's a chemical compound that acts like a shuttle bus. But instead of carrying passengers to the airport, ATP delivers energy to power your cells. Without it, for example, you wouldn't be able to contract your muscles.

But sometimes your body just doesn't produce enough ATP — particularly as you grow older. That's where diet comes in. You'll want to avoid heavily processed foods like deli meat, sweetened cereal, artificially flavored crackers, and frozen pizza. They can increase inflammation, which slows down ATP production. Instead, you'll want to eat vitamin- and mineral-rich whole foods.

Fill your plate with these foods to keep ATP flowing.

- kale, spinach, cauliflower, and Brussels sprouts

- chicken, salmon, and tuna

- egg yolks, nuts, and seeds

> Need more energy? Look no further than beans. These protein-packed pods are loaded with magnesium, which helps convert food into energy. Eat a cup of boiled black beans a day for 30% of your magnesium requirements and 60% of your fiber needs. All that fiber can slow glucose absorption and help steady your blood sugar levels.

Veggies balance blood sugar blues. Feel sleepy an hour or so after a frosty shake and french fries at the drive-thru? Most people do. Fast foods have a high glycemic load (GL) — a measure of how many carbohydrates a food contains and how quickly they will make your blood sugar rise. It's that sugar spike, followed by a sharp drop, that makes you want to nod off. So it makes sense that foods with a low GL would have the opposite effect.

And that's just what researchers found after four weeks of feeding high- and low-GL diets to 82 adults. The people who ate the high-GL diet — think mashed potatoes instead of barley pilaf and white bagels instead of whole-grain bread — scored 26% higher on tests for fatigue.

Add these low-GL foods to keep your blood sugar steady.

- lentils, kidney beans, chickpeas, and soybeans
- cashews and peanuts
- fiber-rich fruits and vegetables, like carrots, green peas, apples, and grapefruit

Tuckered out? Load up on B12 to stay on your feet

You might already know that vitamin B12 deficiency can cause confusion, depression, and memory problems. It can even cause your hands and feet to go numb.

Here's one more to add to the list — fatigue. If you become anemic because you're not getting enough of this important nutrient, you may feel worn out, short of breath, and even dizzy. That's because your red blood cells aren't carrying enough oxygen from your lungs to the rest of your body.

So what can you do? Have your doctor test your vitamin B12 level. If it's low, load up on clams, oysters, and liver — three of the vitamin's best sources. Add variety with nutrient-packed foods like eggs, milk, fortified breakfast cereal, salmon, mackerel, and tuna.

Be aware that some people have problems absorbing B12 from food and supplements. Luckily, you can also get your boost from injections prescribed by your doctor.

There's no fudging the truth — dark chocolate may curb exhaustion

Did you know the Aztecs valued chocolate so much they traded cocoa beans as currency? In fact, their emperor Montezuma II thought so highly of chocolate's fatigue-fighting powers that he once proclaimed, "A cup of this precious drink permits man to walk for a whole day without food."

Some 500 years later, scientists decided to test Montezuma's theory. They discovered that this "food of the gods" may be key in relieving the exhaustion that accompanies chronic fatigue syndrome (CFS), a little-understood disorder that can leave sufferers physically drained for years on end.

British researchers split a small group of CFS patients and gave half of them 15 grams (g) of dark chocolate — containing 85% cocoa — three times a day over eight weeks. That adds up to 45 g a day — the size of a standard Hershey's bar.

The other half ate the same amount of a specially prepared fake chocolate that looked and tasted just like the real McCoy. Then the roles were reversed. Over another eight weeks, participants ate the sweet they hadn't yet consumed.

Sure enough, the people who ate the dark chocolate saw a significant improvement in their fatigue. What's more, they were less depressed and anxious and were better able to engage in daily activities. And when they switched over to the fake fare? Their symptoms worsened.

One possible reason? Dark chocolate is rich in flavonoids, powerful antioxidants that may ease the symptoms of CFS by fighting inflammation and cell damage.

Just make sure you choose the dark kind and balance the extra calories by eating less of other foods.

Eat to beat anemia with a cast-iron plan

What do spoon-shaped fingernails, excessive hair loss, and a hankering to eat paper have in common? They're unusual symptoms of iron-deficiency anemia — a condition that develops when your body doesn't have enough iron to produce hemoglobin. That's the protein that helps your red blood cells carry oxygen.

And the most common signs that something is wrong? Bone-weary fatigue, muscle weakness, and shortness of breath. That makes sense, considering your body needs oxygen to convert food into energy.

Unfortunately, you're more likely to become anemic as you get older. And that can put you at greater risk of falling, longer hospitalizations, and losing your independence.

But iron deficiency isn't an inevitable part of aging. To get your recommended 8 milligrams (mg) a day, try the top iron-rich foods in each of these categories.

- Meats. Eat 3 ounces of pan-fried chicken liver to get 11 mg.

- Shellfish. Chow down on 3 ounces of steamed oysters for 8 mg.

- Legumes. A cup of cooked white beans fetches 7 mg.

- Leafy greens. Munch on 1 cup of cooked spinach to get 6 mg.

It's no yolk: No-prep eggs put a pep in your step

Looking for a morning meal that provides long-lasting energy? Start your day with the incredible, edible egg. Research shows that the protein in eggs helps you avoid the blood sugar peaks and valleys that can make you tired. Eggs are also rich in leucine, an essential amino acid that helps your muscles use energy.

So scramble up this nutritious breakfast. You won't even need a skillet.

- Coat a microwave-safe mug with cooking spray. Blend in an egg with a tablespoon of water — and half a cup of your favorite veggies for an extra nutrient boost — then salt and pepper to taste.

- Microwave on high for 30 seconds. Gently stir. Continue to microwave until egg is almost set, an additional 30 to 45 seconds.

- Serve with whole-grain toast.

Gallstones

Skip the stones with 3 blockbuster nutrients

Half of all women are going to develop gallstones by the time they celebrate their 75th birthday. Think about that for a minute. If 50% of women will get gallstones, that means it could happen to your best friend. Or your sister. Or it could even happen to you. Read on to find out how to protect yourself — and the people you love — from the pain, nausea, and fever sometimes caused by gallstones.

Your gallbladder is a small pear-shaped organ found under the liver on the right side of your abdomen. Its main job is to store bile, an enzyme that helps your body digest fats. When food enters your small intestine, your body releases a hormone that signals the gallbladder to contract and secrete the bile that helps turn fat into energy.

And it's a perfect system, until something goes wrong. Like gallstones. Bile salts, made from cholesterol in the liver, can harden into gallstones that range in size from a grain of sand to about the size of an egg. And if these stones block the flow of bile, you may experience symptoms like pain in your right shoulder or back, abdominal pain, vomiting, and jaundice — a yellowing of the skin and eyes.

High-fiber foods help you stay stone-free. Stop gallstones from building up in your system by boosting both kinds of fiber.

- Soluble fiber — found in foods like oats, barley, nuts, seeds, beans, apples, and blueberries — absorbs bile salts and carries them out of your system.

Eat

Brown rice	Oats
Broccoli	Nuts
Pineapple	Coffee
Strawberries	

Avoid

Foods with saturated fats like whole milk and butter

Commercially baked goods like cakes and pies that contain trans fats

- Insoluble fiber, from whole-wheat bread, brown rice, cauliflower, green beans, and potatoes, speeds food through your digestive tract so bile doesn't have time to collect and form gallstones.

You may be tempted to settle for that pricey fiber supplement you see on store shelves. But experts say whole foods are better at providing the different kinds of fiber and vitamins you need for good health. Stock up on fresh fruits and vegetables instead.

Beat back gallstones with vitamin C. Experts have found that women with higher levels of vitamin C in their blood experience less gallbladder trouble. In fact, one observational study showed that regularly supplementing with vitamin C was linked to a lower risk of gallstones.

You'll find lots of supplements on store shelves that promise to up your C. But you can easily get the recommended amount from real food. Try adding an avalanche of common vitamin C-rich foods to your menu. Are you a veggie lover? Pile on the broccoli, cauliflower, and Brussels sprouts. More of a fruit connoisseur? Pineapples and strawberries fill the bill for you.

Want to avoid gallstones? Better keep an eye on what goes in your stomach. Gallstones are caused by changes in bile, the liquid made by the liver to digest food. Studies show diets high in saturated fats and trans fats cause the bile — which contains mostly cholesterol and fats — to crystallize and form stones.

Healthy fats block the rocks. Although fats often get a bad rap, monounsaturated and polyunsaturated fats are just what the doctor ordered to protect you from gallstones. These good-for-you unsaturated fats help your gallbladder contract and empty on a regular basis, lowering the chance for stones to form.

Get a delicious dose of these fats from olive oil, canola oil, avocados, and even nuts. Wait. Nuts, really? You bet. Harvard researchers found that eating at least 5 ounces of nuts each week lowered the risk of gallstones by 30% in a group of more than 80,000 women.

It's true nuts are fatty, but it's the good fat — the kind that helps to keep bad LDL cholesterol low — so the cholesterol levels in bile stay low, too.

Feel free to harvest a healthy helping of 1 1/2 ounces of nuts like pecans, walnuts, pistachios, cashews, and almonds every day. But remember, nuts are high in calories, so enjoy a handful as a snack instead of chips or cookies. Or add them to salads and sandwiches for a delicious twist to a favorite dish.

Sous vide cooking preserves veggie's vitamin C

To get the most C out of your broccoli, ditch your steamer and pitch your pot. For healthier veggies, scientists want you to try a cooking method called sous vide, a French term that means "under vacuum."

When you cook broccoli in traditional ways, it loses nutrients. Heat damages the veggie's cell walls, allowing vitamin C and water to escape. Sous vide leaves the cell walls mostly intact, so your broccoli stays nutrient-packed and gets more tender.

The only special equipment you'll need for sous vide cooking is an appliance called an immersion circulator, available online or at department stores.

Place your immersion circulator and vacuum-sealed veggies in a container of water and set it for the recommended temperature — usually 183 degrees for broccoli, but check your recipe for suggestions. Cook your broccoli for as little as 15 minutes or as long as 40. Your immersion circulator will heat and circulate the water at a precise, consistent temp to keep your food healthy and delicious.

Brew news: Coffee stalls gallstone buildup

"What goes best with a cup of coffee? Another cup," joked Henry Rollins, an American comedian. And when it comes to preventing gallstones, he's right on the money.

Coffee's perks are well-grounded. Drinking just 1 cup of coffee each day decreases your risk of developing gallstones by 5%. Up your intake by 1 more cup, and you'll see even better results.

Researchers discovered that folks who drink 2 cups of caffeinated coffee every day reduce their risk of gallbladder disease by 11%. Have 3 cups, and your risk drops by 15%. If you're a real coffee buff, you might even indulge in as many as 4 cups a day. If so, your caffeine habit could be the ticket to lower your risk of developing gallstones by nearly 20%. Great news for coffee lovers, but how's it work?

> If coffee's not your cup of tea, wet your whistle with water instead. H2O helps your gallbladder empty so bile can't build up. And that prevents gallstones from forming. Researchers think 2 cups of water, four times a day should keep your gallbladder humming along right as rain.

Stonewall gallstones with a gut reaction. Scientists think it may be the caffeine in coffee that stimulates the contraction of the gallbladder. This helps get rid of the cholesterol-filled bile that can harden into stones. So coffee is good news for preventing gallstones — and for keeping small crystals from turning into bigger ones.

But researchers are stumped. If it were just the caffeine at work, caffeinated sodas or teas would have the same effect. Oops. They don't. So, although caffeine helps, there's a mystery ingredient in coffee that's warding off those stones.

Experts think it may be coffee's magnesium. One study showed that men who got adequate amounts of magnesium in their diets — that's 420 milligrams (mg) per day for men and 320 mg for women — had a 32% lower risk of developing gallstones than their magnesium-deficient peers. More magnesium research is needed, but for now, relax and enjoy a healthy cuppa joe — it's good to the last drop.

Rapid weight loss bumps up gallstone risk

Fast weight loss programs promise that if you eat the right food or use the right supplements, you'll be model-slim in no time. But look out. Those quick-loss plans could leave you with some weighty gallbladder problems.

Being overweight boosts your chances of developing gall-stones, especially for women. Turns out that people who are obese may produce high levels of cholesterol in their bile — even more than the bile can dissolve. And that can mean gallstone trouble.

But losing weight too quickly can make your liver release extra cholesterol into the bile and prevent the gallbladder from emptying properly. Uh-oh.

After studying quick verses slow weight loss in more than 11,000 people, associate professor Jennifer Kuk of York University said, "Given the risk for gallstones with faster weight loss, trying to lose weight at the recommended 1 to 2 pounds per week is the safer option."

Gingivitis

Get rid of gingivitis with the three G's

Ever had red, tender gums that bled when you brushed or flossed? Those are all signs you could have gingivitis. Other symptoms may not be as obvious — like slowly receding gums. Gingivitis is the earliest stage of gum disease, most often caused by the buildup of bacterial plaque between and around your teeth.

Left untreated, gingivitis can worsen and become periodontitis. That's when the bone around your teeth becomes damaged, which could cause your teeth to loosen and even fall out.

If you want to stave off gingivitis, all you have to do is remember the letter "G." Grapefruit, guava, and gazpacho all contain a pigment called lycopene that may act as an antioxidant to guard your gums.

Fruit fortifies your mouth against damage. A small randomized, placebo-controlled clinical trial shows that pairing a lycopene-rich diet with good oral hygiene can be an effective treatment against gingivitis.

The standard dental treatment for scraping tartar and plaque off teeth reduced gingivitis 10% to 20%. But participants who had their teeth cleaned and also took 8 milligrams of lycopene daily showed even greater improvement — nearly 30% in just one week.

Guava and grapefruit can help you out by giving you more lycopene. They're among the fruits highest in this important nutrient. Plus they contain another antioxidant, vitamin C, which can help slow periodontitis. Find out more about how C fights gingivitis in the story *Peppers put the 'p' in 'prevention.'* Make sure grapefruit won't affect your medications before adding it to your diet.

Eat	
Peppers	Tomatoes
Guava	Grapefruit
Grapes	Apples
Peanuts	Black pepper

Avoid
Food and drinks with added sugar

Seeing red on your plate helps your gums. Since lycopene gives many foods their red color, it's no surprise that tomatoes are your best source of lycopene. That's why the third "G" you want to look for is gazpacho. The soup of the summer, this chilled dish is full of tomatoes and tasty vegetables for a refreshing flavor.

Boost the amount of lycopene you get from your tomato recipes, without adding extra tomatoes, by cooking them. Heat processing enhances antioxidant activity. That's why one of the easiest ways to get more lycopene is drinking a glass of tomato juice. Look for options without added sugars, which are linked to inflammation and gum disease.

The dose of lycopene used in the clinical trial was less than the amount you'll find in a whole tomato. In comparison, gazpacho recipes often end up with about three-fourths of a fresh tomato per serving. Plus most recipes call for tomato juice or canned crushed tomatoes, offering more lycopene with every bite.

Kick up the benefits of this classic salad

You may be familiar with the classic Waldorf salad. This variation comes with a trio of ingredients that may fight gingivitis through one super compound called resveratrol.

Found in grapes, apples, and peanuts, resveratrol is great for fending off cavities. And through its anti-inflammatory and antioxidant qualities, experts say it may be a boon for your gum health.

To make four servings of the salad, measure 6 tablespoons of plain yogurt into a large bowl — this is your healthy alternative to mayonnaise. You may want to stir in a bit of honey to sweeten it, then whisk in 1/2 teaspoon of salt and a pinch of black pepper.

Next, chop up two or three apples and toss 'em in. Mix in a cup each of sliced grapes, thinly sliced celery (about three stalks), and peanuts. Serve on a bed of fresh lettuce.

Peppers put the 'p' in 'prevention'

When it comes to your gums, color matters. Too pale may be a sign of anemia, too red could suggest gingivitis. Color makes a difference when picking peppers, too. They don't just taste different — their nutrients vary. And if you want to fight off gingivitis, vitamin C is a big one to look for. Although good dental hygiene, like brushing and flossing, is the first step in preventing gum disease, vitamin C is one of the best nutrients for protecting your gums.

When green doesn't mean "go." Ever wonder why green peppers are more bitter than their warm-colored counterparts, or why you sometimes find spots of a different color on them? Green bell peppers are unripe versions of red, yellow, and orange bell peppers. Because they haven't been on the stem as long, they also have lower amounts of certain nutrients.

For instance, you can get up to twice as much vitamin C in red and yellow bell peppers than green ones. This powerful antioxidant helps fight the inflammation and damage associated with gingivitis.

> Bells aren't the only kind of pepper that can fight gingivitis. Piperine, found in black pepper, is an anti-inflammatory. It helps your body better absorb gingivitis-fighting chemicals like curcumin and lycopene.

Scientists have found that vitamin C may reduce gum bleeding caused by gingivitis. And one recent study revealed that eating more vitamin C may help slow the progression of gum disease. In fact, the researchers say adding more antioxidant-packed fruits and veggies to your diet may help prevent the condition.

Your gums' vast network of influence. Why is controlling gingivitis so important? It doesn't just impact your oral health. Gum disease can affect conditions that seem totally unrelated like heart disease, stroke, and pneumonia. The bacteria in your mouth can spread to other parts of your body, such as your lungs and circulatory system, which is responsible for blood flow.

Diabetes and gum health are also connected. Experts consider diabetes a risk factor for periodontitis, an advanced stage of gum disease. And recent research shows a stronger link between vitamin C and periodontitis for people with diabetes. In one study, vitamin C helped improve gum bleeding in people who had both conditions.

The surprising way gum helps your gums

Like to freshen up your breath with a piece of gum? You may be getting even more benefits than you think if you choose the sugar-free variety.

Chewing gum increases saliva flow in your mouth. That can help clear out any left behind carbohydrates that feed bacteria. Plus it can raise your mouth's pH, combating the acidity that eats away at enamel and causes cavities.

As a study of teens suggests, chewing sugar-free gum may also reduce gingivitis and plaque. Scientists are still researching what gum-chewing routine gives the best result.

Chewing in general may encourage a protective immune response in your gums. A recent animal study showed that chewing triggers the release of Th17 cells, which are part of the immune system and help protect against illness.

Your toothbrush can get covered in bacteria just from sitting near your toilet. Yuck. But that doesn't mean you have to shell out money for a new one every few months. Soak the bristles in white vinegar for 10 minutes to clean them and save yourself a trip to the store — and the doctor's office.

Just remember, chewing gum isn't a substitute for brushing. So don't toss out the toothbrush just yet.

Add this gum-friendly plant to your nightly routine

Ever heard of neem? It's a tree native to India and nearby countries, where it's been used to treat almost every condition under the sun — including gingivitis.

Neem twigs are often used in India as a sort of toothbrush, called a chewing stick. But neem has also been made into other products you're more familiar with.

In one study, participants who used neem-based toothpaste had significantly less severe plaque and gingivitis than those who used conventional toothpaste.

Likely at work is neem's main active component, azadirachtin, which is antimicrobial. It attacks and breaks down bacterial cell walls, killing the threat and stopping the spread of bacteria.

If you're ready for a new way to protect against gingivitis, you can easily purchase neem toothpaste and mouthwash online from places like Walmart, Walgreens, and Amazon.

Gout

DASH your risk for painful attacks with this heart-smart plan

Uh-oh. It's 4 a.m. and your big toe feels prickly and hot. A quick glance down reveals a red bump that's swollen and tender. Soon, even the weight of your bed sheet is too much to bear.

Welcome to the world of gout — a form of arthritis that often flares up at night. The cause? A painful buildup of urate crystals in your joints.

Surprisingly, new research suggests that sticking to a heart-healthy meal plan — the Dietary Approaches to Stop Hypertension (DASH) diet — may lower your risk.

That's according to a large study led by researchers at Harvard Medical School. The team followed the eating habits of more than 44,000 men over a whopping 26 years. None of them had a history of gout at the start of the study.

The scientists scored the people in the study on how closely they followed the DASH diet's emphasis on fruits and vegetables, nuts, beans, whole grains, and low-fat dairy. They also rated how closely their food choices matched the typical Western diet, which is high in red and processed meats, french fries, sweets, and refined grains.

After accounting for known risk factors like age, body mass index, and high blood pressure, the scientists found that higher DASH scores were tied to a lower risk of gout, whereas higher Western-diet scores were linked to a higher risk.

Eat	
Nuts	Beans
Turmeric	Cherries
Whole grains	

Avoid

Processed meats
Alcoholic beverages
Organ meats
Refined grains

Unfortunately, the scientists weren't able to prove cause and effect. But, they say, the DASH diet may be a good all-around approach because it also treats high blood pressure — a condition that affects the majority of gout patients.

In addition, a previous study showed that the DASH eating plan was much better than the Western-style diet in lowering blood levels of uric acid in people who had high concentrations of it. Too much uric acid, after all, is the reason those nasty, needle-shaped urate crystals accumulate in your joints.

The perils of purine — new studies shake up old advice

You might know that Benjamin Franklin invented the lightning rod and bifocals. But few people realize his senior years were marked by repeated attacks of gout. In fact, four men had to carry Franklin in a specially made chair to the Constitutional Convention in Philadelphia.

Why was the founding father so prone to flare-ups? Most likely his love of wine, rich foods, and red meats. They're all loaded with purine, a compound that breaks down into uric acid in your blood.

So you'll want to limit — or avoid — these purine-rich foods to prevent attacks.

- seafood like anchovies, sardines, scallops, mussels, lobster, and shrimp

- bacon, turkey, and organ meats like liver and kidneys

- beef, lamb, and pork

- all types of alcoholic beverages

And while doctors once advised people with gout not to eat vegetables high in purine — mushrooms, beans, peas, asparagus, and spinach, for example — that may no longer be necessary.

A study of the eating habits of more than 600 gout sufferers found that the purine they ate from animal sources raised a much higher risk of a gout flare-up than the purine from plant sources.

The researchers say it's because plant-based foods have less purine than meats and seafood. In addition, the fiber and healthy fats in vegetables may help reduce insulin resistance — a major factor in gout development and attacks.

The results of a more recent study still call for caution. Those researchers say plant-based purine doesn't seem to raise your chances of developing gout. But, they say, you should be cautious with purine-heavy vegetables — or replace them with low-purine alternatives — if you already have gout or advanced kidney disease.

Your best bet? Talk to your doctor before making any changes to your diet.

Fearing future flare-ups? Cherry-bomb 'em

Don't want to join the millions of Americans sidelined by an attack of gout? Reach for a bowl of yummy — and nutritious — cherries.

That's the advice of Boston University researchers who examined the diets of more than 630 gout patients for a year, paying special attention to their diets during the two days before a gout attack.

- They discovered that those who had eaten cherries over a two-day period ran a 35% lower risk of a flare-up than those who didn't eat the fruit. The magic number of cherries to avoid an attack? Participants saw benefits with up to three servings over the two days — an average of about 15 to 18 cherries a day.

Cherries not in season? No worries. Researchers saw a significant reduction in gout flare-ups among participants who took 1 tablespoon of concentrated cherry juice — equal to 45 to 60 cherries — twice a day over four months.

- Results were even stronger for the people who ate cherries and took allopurinol, a medication used to treat gout and kidney stones. Their risk of gout attacks dropped 75% compared to periods with no cherries or drug.

So what's so special about cherries? They're rich in anthocyanins, pigments that give fruits and vegetables their red, blue, and purple colors. Anthocyanins may also combat inflammation, which is linked to the painful swelling that occurs when urate crystals form in your joints.

In addition, previous studies have linked cherries to reduced levels of uric acid in the blood. That's important, because a buildup of the compound often leads to gout. Researchers aren't exactly sure how cherries do it, but they say the fruit may help lower your body's production of uric acid or assist your kidneys in filtering it from your blood.

Buy and store cherries like a pro

Ever wonder about the origins of the Bing cherry? It's the brainchild of an unlikely duo who became friends on an Oregon fruit orchard in the late 1800s. One of them was the owner, Seth Lewelling. The other was his Chinese foreman, Ah Bing. Once their new variety of cherry took fruit, Lewelling honored Bing by naming it after him.

Today, Bing cherries are probably the most popular sweet cherry in the supermarket. But before you buy, look for shiny, plump, and firm cherries that have bright green stems attached — they're fresher and may not go bad as fast.

Once home, store them unwashed in the fridge either between layers of paper towel or in an airtight plastic bag. The cherries will keep for at least a week. Rinse before eating.

Cherries also freeze well. Just rinse, pat dry, and seal in an airtight plastic bag.

Turmeric: Go for the gold with this anti-inflammatory spice

South Asians have used turmeric — the pungent, earthy-sweet spice that gives curry powder its distinct golden color — for centuries to treat health problems like rheumatism and fatigue. And now scientists in China have discovered that a substance in turmeric may reduce gout-related inflammation.

Researchers in a recent study gave a group of mice the main active ingredient in turmeric — curcumin. Other mice didn't receive any. An hour later, the scientists injected urate crystals into the paws and ankles of both groups. Sure enough, the mice dosed with curcumin had a lot less swelling than the other group.

According to the scientists, curcumin may prevent a protein — nuclear factor-kappa B — from triggering an inflammatory response in your body.

Of course, more studies are needed to see if humans get equally beneficial results. But it's never too early to add this healthy spice to your diet.

- Add a pinch or two to rice, soups, and scrambled eggs.

- Toss it on vegetables before roasting.

- Sprinkle over popcorn.

- Add to salad dressing.

Headaches & Migraines

Secret to stopping the pain before it starts

Don't wait until your head is throbbing to change up your diet. You can stop some headaches before they even happen just by eating the right foods. Certain ones are considered "pain safe" because they almost never contribute to conditions like headaches and migraines.

How do you know what type of headache you have? If you feel a dull, squeezing sensation in your forehead, scalp, temples, or neck you likely have a tension headache. Pain on one side of your head or a stabbing feeling behind your eye are signs of a cluster headache.

Both of these are primary headaches, meaning they aren't caused by another condition. You can also have secondary headaches which have underlying causes, for instance, sleep apnea.

On the other hand, you'll probably have other symptoms if you have a migraine. You may experience heightened sensitivity to sound, light, or smells; feel nauseated; or see an aura of light. You'll usually feel a moderate to severe, throbbing pain on one side of your head, which gets worse at the slightest movement.

Veg out the healthy way. In a study of adults with migraines reported in the *Journal of Headache and Pain*, researchers found that a plant-based diet can reduce migraine pain. The participants ate a low-fat, vegan diet that removed potential triggers like meat and dairy.

Eat

Broccoli	Squash
Rice	Salmon
Chives	Bran
Ginger	Feverfew tea
Sunflower seeds	
Pumpkin seeds	

Avoid

Processed meats

Pickled and fermented foods

Aged cheeses

Caffeine

Alcohol

Artificial sweeteners

- Although scientists aren't exactly sure what causes migraines, they believe inflammation and blood vessel expansion, called vasodilation, play critical roles. Plant foods are high in antioxidants and anti-inflammatory compounds that can combat these problems.

- The study's participants may have benefitted from weight loss. Past research shows migraines have improved with weight loss, which can occur when you switch to a plant-based diet.

- Folate may also be a factor in fighting migraines. B vitamins, including folate, reduce homocysteine levels in your body, which decreases migraine symptoms. An Australian study found that eating more folate lowered migraine frequency in women who experienced auras. Eating vegetables is an easy way to add folate to your diet. Spinach and turnip greens are packed with it and pain-safe to boot.

Eat well to feel your best. Focus on swapping processed and fast foods for healthier choices, and see if that helps keep migraines away. In a recent Iranian study in the journal *Headache*, women with infrequent migraines had an overall better diet than those with chronic migraines.

Raise the quality of yours by following the government's dietary guidelines and sticking to pain-safe foods when you can. Cooked green, orange, and yellow vegetables — like broccoli, carrots, and squash — are all unlikely to give you headache trouble. Besides veggies, pain-free foods include rice and cooked or dried noncitrus fruits.

One dangerous cause of headaches is hypertension. You may not realize you have high blood pressure since there usually aren't any symptoms. But if your pressure reaches 180/120, you could experience a severe headache, along with other symptoms like dizziness and blurred vision. If you suspect your blood pressure is high, get medical attention immediately.

A+ action plan to eliminate your headaches

Overhaul your typical meal plans and start fresh with an elimination diet. You'll ditch all the food that makes your head feel like it's cracking open and figure out which ones are at the root of your pain.

First, eliminate all potential triggers from your diet for about four weeks. You'll want to avoid the dirty dozen, certain grains like barley and rye, and other foods. Check the eat and avoid box at the beginning of this chapter for where to start. You may want to ask your doctor or dietitian for help.

Gradually add the potential triggers back into your diet — no more than one food per day. Keep a record of the food you eat and any headaches or migraines you have so you can find your personal triggers. Avoid those foods in the future, and eat everything else with peace of mind.

Starve a migraine of these trigger foods

Does it seem like your head hurts every time you eat meat? Are you the only friend who thinks chocolate is a head-splitter? It's hard to be on good terms with your food when you don't know if it will feel like a cranium crusher later.

Many foods contain compounds that could trigger a migraine through inflammation or by widening your blood vessels, called vasodilation. Here are a few you may need to avoid.

Say bye-bye to pain provokers. Twelve common foods that trigger migraines — dubbed the "dirty dozen" — are meat, chocolate, dairy, eggs, citrus fruits, wheat, nuts and peanuts, tomatoes, onions, corn, apples, and bananas. You may want to keep a food diary to see if a migraine flares after you eat any of those. The following compounds can also give you grief.

- Tyramine is often linked to migraines and is commonly found in aged cheeses, products with monosodium glutamate (MSG), processed meats, and pickled and fermented foods. Scientists have found that meat products in general have inflammatory properties, so cutting them from your diet may help your headaches.

- Caffeine is both a blessing and a curse when it comes to headaches. Caffeine may lower your risk of a headache by improving the effect of painkillers and restricting blood flow — the opposite of vasodilation. But ever faced withdrawal? If you cut caffeine cold turkey, you may feel like you've dropped your empty coffee mug on your head. Be selective about your beverage of choice. Doctors advise drinking no more caffeine than 3 cups of coffee's worth per day. Keep in mind that even decaf coffee has some caffeine, and so does chocolate and some teas.

- Histamine is a word you may associate with allergies, but this compound may play a role in migraines, too. Studies report that it could cause and worsen headaches. The exact reason for this isn't known, but it may be a result of vasodilation or inflammation. Foods such as fish, aged cheese, and vegetables like spinach and eggplant all contain histamine.

Can alcohol give you more than a hangover? Like a number of foods, alcohol contains histamines that may hike up a headache. Since it's a vasodilator, it makes your blood vessels expand, which can lead to inflammation and pain. Alcohol also may contain other compounds that cause problems, like tyramine and sulfites.

Familiar with sweet, salty, sour, and bitter? What about the newest base flavor on the block called umami? It's associated with a savory, meaty taste — even in veggies. A recent study suggests umami can cause migraines. MSG is a source of umami, so if it's a trigger for you, that may be the reason.

Although some studies have reported alcohol, especially red wine, to be a trigger, results have been inconsistent. If you enjoy an occasional glass of wine, instead of eliminating it from your diet, test it for yourself, and see if you get negative side effects.

Sugar substitutes are not such a sweet idea. You may have switched to an artificial sweetener to cut back on calories or tooth decay, but these nonnutritive choices could be the root of your headache troubles. Both the American Migraine Foundation and the Mayo Clinic say additives like aspartame may trigger migraines.

In a recent Canadian study of young teens and children, 13 of the 100 participants had aspartame-triggered headaches, showing it does affect some people. If you're a diet soda fan or add artificial sweeteners to your coffee, try cutting back or eliminating them to see if it helps.

Herbal relief from your worst headaches

You woke up with your head throbbing. You know you should take your migraine medication, but you dread the side effects that make you feel even worse. What if you could lessen or even stop the pain without the nasty backlash? Here are two herbs that can improve your headaches the natural way.

Feverfew goes above and beyond to fight migraines. It's not often that a product can do even more than its name suggests. That's why feverfew is a superstar herb. Effective not only against fevers, it's traditionally been used to treat aches from head to stomach and has been especially successful against migraines.

- An aromatic and bushy plant, feverfew makes a helpful, although slightly bitter, tea. Its hydrating power is a great bonus since drinking too little water can give you a headache, too. If it makes your mouth feel dry or irritated, try using more water and fewer leaves or steeping it for a shorter time.

- Not big on hot drinks? Feverfew is available as a supplement, either alone or with other helpful nutrients. In a recent Italian study, scientists combined feverfew and other compounds into a "nutraceutical" supplement to combat headaches. The extra nutrients included magnesium, riboflavin, CoQ10, and an extract from a plant called green chiretta. After four months, this treatment significantly reduced the frequency and pain intensity of the participants' tension headaches and migraines.

Scientists think feverfew's anti-migraine activity is related to several factors, including its ability to block nitric-oxide synthesis and to release serotonin into your system.

How much do you need? Anywhere from 50 milligrams (mg) to a little over 100 mg per day is common in studies, but your doctor may recommend more.

A typical over-the-counter supplement includes 380 mg of standardized feverfew. Check the label to be sure it contains at least 0.2% parthenolide, its active ingredient.

Get to the root of your migraine problem with ginger. Taking an herb that is as effective as a prescription drug may sound crazy, but it's true. When it comes to headaches, you could save hundreds with this homegrown solution.

Ginger's healing power can fix everything from motion sickness to vertigo. And against migraines, ginger works as well as the medication sumatriptan — without the side effects.

Both sumatriptan and ginger improved pain symptoms in a study published in *Phytotherapy Research*. The participants who took sumatriptan experienced side effects including dizziness and heartburn. But the only problem the ginger users faced was indigestion.

Just drop around 1/8 of a teaspoon of ginger into your glass of water at the first sign of a migraine to absorb the great results.

Get ginger ready in a snap

You've brought the perfect piece of ginger home to spice up your next migraine-fighting meal. Here's how to ready and store it for no-fuss prep.

Ginger is knotted which makes it hard to get the skin off with a peeler or a knife. An easy trick? Use a spoon instead. Grip the spoon firmly at the base of its bowl and, holding the concave side downward, use the tip to scrape off the skin. Only peel as much as you're going to use. The leftovers will store better with the outer layer still attached.

When you're ginger-ed out for the day, put it in a freezer bag and squeeze out all the air. Then put it in your refrigerator's crisper drawer to keep it fresh for three weeks. Or leave it in your freezer for up to six months.

Next time it will be even more painless. Frozen ginger grates with ease and makes cleaning up a breeze.

Fight back with a trio of powerhouse nutrients

Aspirin may be your go-to for pain, but you don't have to rely on it to banish headaches. Making sure you get these nutrients in your diet could be enough to ward them off.

Fight inflammation with vitamin D and calcium. Scientists believe anywhere from 45% to 100% of people who get migraines and headaches are low in vitamin D. In fact, that deficiency may help kick-start your headaches. It may also increase the frequency and severity of migraine attacks.

Supplementing your diet with vitamin D may reduce both of these negative effects. Because it's an antioxidant and anti-inflammatory, this nutrient fights inflammation in your nervous system that could lead to — and worsen — head pain.

Low calcium levels may play a role as well. Vitamin D is essential to calcium absorption, so lacking both nutrients may impact how often you suffer from migraines and how intense they are.

Make your life easy by eating foods high in both nutrients, like cheddar and Swiss cheese. If dairy triggers your headaches, canned salmon knocks vitamin D and calcium levels out of the park, too.

Migraines meet their match with magnesium. When a group of researchers analyzed multiple studies on taking magnesium, they found the supplements can significantly reduce the number of migraines you get. They've also reported that taking magnesium can make pain levels more tolerable.

The National Institutes of Health recommends 420 milligrams (mg) of magnesium per day for men and 320 mg for women. Since supplements above daily recommended amounts are common, use them under your doctor's supervision.

Looking for a way to add magnesium to your meals? Foods like rice and wheat bran, chives, and pumpkin and sunflower seeds are all packed with it and ready to knock out your headaches.

Heart disease

Beat back cardiac concerns with 4 pantry staples

Your heart beats around 100,000 times a day, pumping 2,000 gallons of blood through your circulatory system. That's a lot of hard work — without a single break — to keep you up and running. So why not return the favor by lowering your risk of heart disease?

You probably know your diet plays a major role in determining the health of your ticker. Here's the science behind four foods that help ward off the leading causes of heart disease. And the best part? They're probably already in your kitchen.

Take time for tea and get cleaner arteries. Research suggests that drinking almost 4 cups of black tea a day over four weeks may boost blood flow and improve artery function in people with heart disease.

Atherosclerosis, the buildup of plaques within the walls of the arteries, occurs when the endothelial cells — the ones that line the interior surface of your blood vessels — stop working properly. Black tea improves how well those cells do their job, which may reverse problems that could lead to clogged arteries.

So how did black tea do it? The researchers weren't 100% sure, but say it could be linked to black tea's powerful antioxidants — substances that fight off harmful rogue molecules looking to damage your cells.

Nosh on nuts to balance your cholesterol. Walnuts, almonds, and hazelnuts. Just pick your

Eat	
Black tea	Guava
Garlic	Flaxseed
Fish	Blueberries
Cherries	Avocado
Tomatoes	Apples
Nuts	Broccoli sprouts

Avoid
Coconut oil

Fatty foods like butter and bacon

favorite. Spanish scientists found that adding a daily handful of these nuts to the fruit- and vegetable- rich Mediterranean diet works better than adding more olive oil in lowering your chances of metabolic syndrome — a cluster of risk factors that increase your likelihood of heart disease.

All it took was 1/4 cup of mixed nuts a day over one year for people to see improvements in their cholesterol. The researchers say the results are due to the large amounts of unsaturated fats in nuts.

Sweeten with honey to battle blood clots. People have used honey to treat wounds for thousands of years. Science now suggests you can also heal your heart with honey.

Researchers believe honey's powerful antioxidants help soften arteries and reduce excess clotting. These natural compounds are also linked to lower levels of low-density lipoprotein (LDL) — the bad choles- terol — that forms into sticky plaques and can clog your arteries.

Studies show that darker varieties of honey have the most antioxidants.

Grate garlic to keep blood pressure in check. Experts recently reviewed numerous studies and found evidence that suggests this simple seasoning can lower your blood pressure and cholesterol.

Scientists believe garlic increases your body's production of nitric oxide, a molecule that relaxes the inner muscles of your blood vessels so that they dilate. This makes it easier for your heart to pump blood and lowers your blood pressure.

Garlic also contains an enzyme thought to block the production of cholesterol. But the little bulb's mighty powers don't stop there.

Garlic may also help prevent blood clots by keeping platelets from clumping together. That's why it could be dangerous to eat it if you're taking blood thinners. If that's the case, talk to your doctor before adding garlic to your diet.

Face the flax — a little seed with mighty powers

Flaxseed is such a nutritional powerhouse that in the eighth century Charlemagne passed laws requiring his subjects to eat them.

The medieval king of the Franks and Lombards may have been on to something. In a modern-day study of 50 people with high cholesterol, those who ate 2 tablespoons of roasted flaxseed powder every day for three months had lower LDL and total cholesterol numbers — and higher levels of high-density lipoprotein, the "good" cholesterol — than those who didn't eat flaxseed.

Experts think this change is caused by alpha linolenic acid, an omega-3 fatty acid known for its heart perks, and polyphenols called lignans.

But the benefits don't stop there. Besides besting high cholesterol, flaxseed also lowers blood pressure and protects against cancer. That's pretty amazing in itself, but this miracle healer also fights arthritis, stomach disorders, and mental problems.

Angling for a healthy heart? Reel in the virtues of fish oil

Americans spend more than $1 billion a year on over-the-counter fish oil. That's enough to send 5,395 students to Harvard University for four years. Why all the interest in fish oil? It's loaded with omega-3 fatty acids — a healthy fat that could help you ward off heart attacks and strokes, and fight depression, diabetes, and cancer.

Taking a standard fish oil supplement containing 360 milligrams of omega-3 fatty acids twice a day for a week gives you the same amount of omega-3 you'd get from eating two 3.5-ounce servings of fatty fish a week. That's the amount of fish the American Heart Association recommends you eat.

Of course, getting your omega-3 fatty acids from food is better than getting them from a supplement. After all, supplements don't provide all the nutrients and fiber you get from a balanced diet. But for seniors who don't like fish, supplements are something to consider. Here's why.

VITAL fish oil cuts heart attack risk. Researchers at Brigham and Women's Hospital recently completed a multiyear study of nearly 26,000 healthy adults age 50 and older without a history of heart disease.

Dubbed the Vitamin D and Omega-3 Trial (VITAL), the scientists gave some of the participants a daily fish oil supplement containing 1 gram of omega-3 fatty acids. That's about the amount you'd find in 1.5 ounces, or less than half a serving, of cooked salmon. Others took a placebo containing olive oil each day.

- Sure enough, the group using the fish oil supplement had a 28% lower risk of heart attack compared with those taking the placebo.

- Volunteers accustomed to eating less than 1 1/2 servings of fish a week and African American participants saw the best results.

"The results indicate that people with low dietary intake of fish will likely obtain a heart benefit from omega-3 fatty acid supplementation," says Dr. JoAnn Manson, lead author of the study.

While the supplements show promise in preventing heart attacks, the researchers found that 1 gram of omega-3 fish oil had no effect on the risk of stroke.

Talk to your doctor before taking fish oil supplements. They can increase the effects of blood thinners and medicine used to treat high blood pressure — putting your health in danger. Fish oil may also reduce the effectiveness of cancer drugs.

Fact or fraud: Is coconut oil good for you?

The promises made by coconut oil enthusiasts have cholesterol-conscious folks confused. Is it truly an awesome oil — or just a fatty fad? Here's what the experts say.

- Does it lower bad LDL cholesterol? No. In a small recent study, women ate about 2 tablespoons of either coconut oil or safflower oil daily for four weeks. Coconut oil actually raised LDL levels significantly more than safflower oil.

- Does it raise good HDL cholesterol? Yes. In another recent study, volunteers ate 3 1/2 tablespoons of either coconut oil, olive oil, or butter every day for four weeks to find out which raised HDL the most. Coconut oil won.

But raising HDL doesn't necessarily make coconut oil healthy. The American Heart Association advises against using coconut oil because it raises LDL, a major cause of heart disease.

"Don't eat it," says Dr. Stephen Kopecky in a Mayo Clinic Minute feature. "It really does raise your bad cholesterol."

High-dose omega-3 REDUCEs strokes. A new study suggests that high doses of eicosapentaenoic acid (EPA) — a type of omega-3 fatty acid found in fish oil — can help prevent strokes in high-risk people. That's what researchers working on the Reduction of Cardiovascular Events with Ethyl–Intervention Trial (REDUCE-IT) found after tracking the health of nearly 8,200 middle-aged adults and seniors on statins.

The participants had normal cholesterol levels but elevated triglycerides — a type of fat found in the blood that's linked to an increased risk of stroke and heart attack.

Half of the volunteers received a daily 4-gram dose of icosapent ethyl — a pure prescription form of the omega-3 fatty acid EPA. The high dose of EPA in the prescription medication is similar to the amount you'd get after eating more than 20 servings of fish. The rest of the volunteers took a placebo.

- The people taking the supplement were 25% less likely to have a first-time heart event, such as stroke, heart attack, or chest pain called angina, compared to the control group receiving a placebo.

- The odds of experiencing a second event went down by 32%, and a third event by 31%. The risk of having four or more events was cut nearly in half.

The scientists conducting the study say more research is needed before they can explain how EPA lowered the risk of stroke and heart attack.

Avoiding the produce aisle? These fruits will encourage a change of heart

Sour grapes, top banana, bad apple, plum job — Americans toss a lot of fruit into their conversations. And why not? Most fruits are low in fat, sodium, and calories. They're also a key source of essential nutrients like potassium, folate, fiber, and vitamin C.

And some may even lower your risk of heart disease. That's because fruits contain phytochemicals, compounds that act as antioxidants and fight inflammation.

Blueberries boost blood-vessel function. Just 1 cup of blueberries a day can strengthen your blood vessels and raise your HDL (good) cholesterol. That's what British scientists discovered in a brand-new, six-month study of this flavorful fruit's effects on 115 overweight and obese seniors.

All of the volunteers had metabolic syndrome — a condition that increases your risk of heart disease because of factors like elevated blood pressure, excess fat around the waist, and high blood sugar.

The researchers divided the seniors into groups. Some of them ate 1 cup of freeze-dried blueberries a day. The rest ate just 1/2 cup of the same or a placebo.

- At the end of the trial, those who ate a full cup of blueberries saw their risk of heart disease drop by up to 15% compared to the placebo group.

- Eating 1/2 cup of blueberries didn't produce the same results, suggesting that obese, high-risk adults may need more anthocyanins — a type of antioxidant that gives red and blue fruits their rich coloring — to get the same health benefits.

Chow down on cherries to cut LDL cholesterol levels. The tiny cherry, containing more than 17 phytochemicals, appears to work like a charm in clearing away artery-clogging plaque better than vitamin supplements.

A small, 12-week University of Delaware study of healthy seniors showed just how good these tasty treats are for your ticker.

- Participants who drank 2 cups of tart cherry juice a day experienced significant drops in their LDL cholesterol — the kind that builds up on the walls of your blood vessels and can block blood flow — compared with a control group who drank the same amount of unsweetened cherry-flavored Kool-Aid.

- What's more, the cherry juice drinkers also experienced improvements in their systolic blood pressure — a measure of the force of blood against your artery walls when your heart beats.

And the reason behind the results? The researchers cite all the antioxidant and anti-inflammatory properties in tart cherry juice's phytochemicals — anthocyanins included.

Flush out clogged arteries with watermelon

The best time to pick a watermelon is just after its underbelly has turned from white to pale yellow. It's just one interesting fact about this sweet summertime fruit that attacks athero-sclerosis, bashes body fat, and clobbers cholesterol.

University of Kentucky researchers discovered the health benefits after three months of feeding two groups of mice a diet high in saturated fat. One set of mice drank 2% water-melon juice while the other had water that matched the carbohydrate content of the watermelon juice.

The mice that drank the watermelon juice gained less weight, had lower LDL cholesterol, and less plaque in their arteries. The study's authors say watermelon is a rich source of the amino acid citrulline, which may be responsible for this hefty fruit's "hearty" benefits.

Rise and dine with 3 hearty-healthy power foods

Never had the opportunity to eat huevos rancheros? Qué lástima — what a shame! Rancher's eggs is a traditional Mexican breakfast — fried eggs over a warm tortilla served with zesty tomatoes, seasoned black beans, and creamy avocado — that has earned an enthusiastic following north of the border.

No big surprise there, considering the ingredients are tasty, filling, and packed with nutrients. Here's why these foods help keep your heart in fighting form.

Eggs deliver hard-boiled antioxidants. Historically, eggs took quite the beating when it came to heart health. That's because a large egg contains 210 milligrams of cholesterol — some 70% of your recommended daily allowance.

But experts now believe that foods high in saturated fats — not cholesterol — encourage your liver to make more LDL cholesterol than it otherwise would.

And eggs are a rich source of lutein and zeaxanthin, two antioxidants that may protect against heart disease.

Harvard Medical School researchers say one egg a day — the amount recommended by the American Heart Association — is safe for most people not at risk for cardiovascular disease. Just don't eat them with fatty foods like butter, bacon, and muffins.

Hot off the vine — tomatoes trim LDL. A small study of nearly 60 people with type 2 diabetes found that just two glasses of tomato juice a day boost LDL's resistance to the harmful effects of oxidation.

Oxidized LDL, cholesterol damaged by chemical interactions with free radicals, is the kind most likely to lead to hardened arteries, heart attacks, and strokes. But lycopene — the pigment in tomatoes that give them their red color — may help prevent this dangerous cholesterol from forming.

In a separate but similar study, scientists gave 481 Japanese adults unlimited amounts of unsalted tomato juice to drink over a year. Most of the participants drank a little less than a cup a day.

At the end of the study, the volunteers who had previously been at risk for heart disease saw large drops in their blood pressure and LDL numbers.

Avocado gets an "A" for plaque prevention. Penn State researchers have found that eating an avocado a day may protect your good cholesterol and fight the bad, artery-clogging kind.

The study recruited 45 overweight and obese adults who followed an average American diet for two weeks. Then, in no particular order, they each completed five weeks of a low-fat diet, a moderate-fat diet, and a moderate-fat diet with a daily avocado.

- After five weeks on the avocado diet, participants had significantly lower levels of oxidized LDL than when they started the study and after completing the low- and moderate-fat diets.

- They also had higher levels of lutein, which may have prevented the LDL from being oxidized.

"Avocados are really high in healthy fats, carotenoids — which are important for eye health — and other nutrients," says Penny Kris-Etherton, distinguished professor of nutrition and author of the study. "They are such a nutrient-dense package, and I think we're just beginning to learn about how they can improve health," she says.

Rock the guac — eat your way to health with smart avocado swaps

Avocados are loaded with fiber, potassium, and healthy fats, making this one-ingredient swap better for your heart than less healthy traditional options.

- Use avocado instead of mayo to bind together the ingredients of chicken, tuna, and egg salads. Or add a drop of olive oil to mashed avocado and spread on your sandwiches in place of mayo.

- Like to add a dollop of sour cream to your soup, baked potato, or taco? You'll get the same creamy consistency with avocado.

- Next time you bake a cake or brownies, substitute half the butter in your recipe with an equal amount of pureed avocado. Lower the oven temperature by 25% to prevent over-browning.

- Trying to stay away from dairy? Nix the cheese in favor of avocados. They're great for topping off sandwiches, salads, and even burgers.

Focus on fiber — a whip-smart way to cut cholesterol

Think you're eating enough fiber? You might want to reconsider. Fewer than 5 in 100 Americans meet their recommended daily intake — for seniors, that's 30 grams for men and 21 grams for women.

Now might be the best time to take a second look at roughage — the portion of plant-based foods your body doesn't break down during digestion. That's because soluble fiber — the kind that mixes with water to form a gel-like substance — does a lot more than keep your body's "plumbing" in good working order.

Soluble fiber also sponges up fats and cholesterol in your small intestine, making sure they get excreted instead of absorbed into your bloodstream. That helps keep your LDL cholesterol and total cholesterol numbers in check, and lowers your risk of heart disease and stroke.

Why not add some of these fun, fiber-filled superfoods to your diet?

Bet on apples. Here's proof this amazing fruit can help lower your cholesterol. In a Florida State University study, 160 women between the ages of 45 and 65 were divided into two groups. The first ate a little less than a cup of dried apples every day for a year, while the second ate dried prunes instead.

One of the researchers, professor Dr. Bahram Arjmandi, was surprised by the results. "Incredible changes in the apple-eating women happened by six months," he says. "They experienced a 23% decrease in LDL cholesterol." Not only that, the apple eaters' HDL numbers climbed 4%.

Dig into konjac. Elephant yam, devil's tongue, and snake palm. Strange nicknames for the heart-healthy plant called konjac (pronounced cognac), a cholesterol-fighting food popular in Asian dishes.

Scientists analyzed the results of 12 studies on konjac and found that the fiber extract — glucomannan — in konjac root has the power to lower your LDL up to 10%. And just 3 grams a day — that's three 1,000-milligram capsules — did the trick.

Glucomannan is available as a supplement in capsule or powder form. Just be sure to follow the directions on the package. You can also enjoy konjac root in konnyaku cake, which is similar to tofu, or in shirataki noodles, also known as "miracle" noodles.

Go for guava. Want to wash artery-clogging LDL right out of your body? A small study of medical students in India found that those who ate 14 ounces of peeled guava fruit a day — about two large guavas — had significant drops in their LDL, triglycerides, and total cholesterol after six weeks.

This delicious fruit may work double duty when it comes to your heart health. Along with its ample supply of soluble fiber, the researchers say antioxidants in guava pulp may also prevent cell damage linked to atherosclerosis.

Psyllium has been shown to lower LDL cholesterol levels by up to 13% and cut blood sugar levels by nearly 20%. And here's more good news. A recent analysis of 28 psyllium trials found that 2 teaspoons of the fiber supplement a day reduces other lipid markers of heart disease as well.

Oddly enough, volunteers who ate the same amount of unpeeled guava saw their total cholesterol, triglycerides, and LDL rise. One possible reason? Magnesium in the peel may have activated enzymes that help the body absorb and digest fats.

High cholesterol cropping up? Sow the benefits of sprouts

Remember the Ch-Ch-Ch-Chia Pet television commercials of the 1980s? Just cover a terra cotta figurine with moist chia seeds and wait for sprouts to form a grass-like carpet of fur. Sure was a fun way to develop a green thumb.

Chia Pets eventually became such a popular gift — more than 15 million sold — that there's one in a time capsule at the American Museum of Natural History in New York.

Of course, you wouldn't want to eat the sprouts growing from your Chia Pet — the seeds don't go through the same safety checks as ones sold for eating. But sprouts sold in supermarkets make a great addition to any meal. And why not? They're low in calories and rich in fiber and other nutrients.

Certain sprouts may even lower your risk of heart disease.

Broccoli sprouts put LDL on notice. A group of Japanese researchers may have discovered a secret for better cholesterol numbers.

- They found that LDL and total cholesterol dropped like a rock in men who ate 3 1/2 ounces of broccoli sprouts a day for one week.

- Women in the small study, meanwhile, showed increases in HDL cholesterol.

And in a separate trial, people with type 2 diabetes who ate a little more than 1/4 ounce of broccoli sprout powder per day over one month saw an 18.7% drop in triglyceride levels and significantly higher HDL numbers.

Lentil sprouts target triglycerides. Iranian researchers divided overweight and obese volunteers with type 2 diabetes into two groups over eight weeks. One group ate a little more than 3/4 cup of lentil sprouts a day. The other didn't eat any sprouts. Both groups were asked not to change their diets or level of activity.

At the end of the study, those who ate the lentil sprouts experienced increases in their HDL numbers and decreases in both triglycerides and oxidized LDL cholesterol.

And the reasons behind the findings?

- Researchers believe the phytonutrients in broccoli and lentil sprouts may bind with bile acids, lowering the amount of cholesterol absorbed into your bloodstream.

- Both broccoli and lentil sprouts are loaded with heart-healthy antioxidants.

Quash doubts about sprouts with these safety tips

Unlike other fresh produce, sprouts grow from seeds and beans under warm and humid conditions. Unfortunately, that's the same environment in which bacteria — including *Salmonella* and *E. coli* — flourish. Eating contaminated sprouts can lead to food poisoning, with severe symptoms that include nausea, vomiting, and diarrhea.

That's why it's important to be careful when shopping for this healthy treat. Buy sprouts when they're crisp, and keep them refrigerated after purchasing. Never eat sprouts that look slimy or discolored. And be sure to wash them under running water before eating or cooking.

The Food and Drug Administration says children, older adults, pregnant women, and people with weakened immune systems should avoid eating raw sprouts. Instead, roast them in the oven until crisp and brown, or add them to soups, stews, and stir-fries.

Heartburn

Spurn the burn: Easy-to-stomach tactics for cutting acid indigestion

Does your game-day snack of zesty Cajun-style chicken wings come with an unwelcome side order of heartburn? If so, you're not alone. Some 60 million Americans experience heartburn — a telltale sign that stomach acid has backed up into your esophagus — at least once a month.

That burning feeling in your chest or throat isn't only painful. It can be downright dangerous. Repeated contact with acid can damage your esophagus — the pipe that carries food from the back of your throat to your stomach — and cause it to develop ulcers, scar tissue, and even cancer. That's because the inner lining of your gullet doesn't have the same protective layer of mucus as your tummy.

So if you're prone to heartburn, you might consider steering clear of common triggers like spicy chili, coffee, raw onions, and orange juice. That's because the foods you eat have an enormous impact on the production of acid in your stomach — and where it goes next. Here's what the research says.

Fatty foods fan unhealthy flames.

Ever hear of gastrosophageal reflux disease (GERD)? It's the technical term for mild acid reflux that occurs at least twice a week, or moderate to severe acid reflux that happens at least once a week.

Scientists were curious about the role nutrition plays in developing GERD. So they followed the eating habits of 371 employees at the Houston VA

Eat

Turmeric	Apples
Pears	Artichokes
Split peas	Oats
Lentils	Water

Avoid

Triggers like fatty, spicy, and fried foods

Table salt

Peppermint tea

Medical Center over a year, carefully examining the amount of vitamins, minerals, carbohydrates, fat, and protein they consumed.

The researchers discovered that overweight volunteers who ate a diet high in fats — particularly the unhealthy saturated kind — ran a significantly higher risk of having GERD and erosive esophagitis, a condition where the inner lining of your gullet becomes inflamed and swollen.

Experts believe high-fat fare — like fast food, fried food, processed meats, and fatty snacks and salad dressings — relax the lower esophageal sphincter, a protective ring of muscle that's supposed to keep stomach acid from leaching into your gullet.

> Some say it's bad luck to spill salt. But shaking it on your food? A study of 25,562 adults in a Norwegian public health survey found that those who added table salt to their meals ran a 70% higher risk of acid reflux than those who never did so.

Mediterranean menu routs reflux. Researchers saw promising results in a recent review of the medical histories of 184 people suffering from laryngopharyngeal reflux, a type of reflux where stomach acid washes up into the throat.

Six weeks of eating a plant-based Mediterranean diet and drinking alkaline water — a type of water that's less acidic than what pours from the tap — lowered symptoms as well as, if not better than, proton-pump inhibitors. Those are the drugs used to lower the amount of acid made by glands in the lining of your stomach.

The researchers believe alkaline water and the special diet help neutralize or lower the activity of pepsin, a digestive enzyme that causes inflammation when it seeps into the throat with stomach acid.

The benefits of the plant-based menu don't stop there. Many of the people who stuck to the diet of mostly fruits, vegetables, grains, and nuts also lost weight and saw improvements in their blood pressure and cholesterol levels.

Switch it up with a fresh take on turmeric

Have a recipe calling for turmeric? Don't run for the spice rack just yet. A fresher option may be sitting right next to its knobby-jointed cousin — ginger root — in the produce aisle.

At first glance, turmeric root may not look like much. But under its dull brown peel lies bright orange flesh eager to add a peppery edge to your next meal.

When preparing fresh turmeric, wear kitchen gloves to avoid getting orange-yellow stains on your fingers. Scrape off the paper-thin peel with a spoon. Grate the root into marinades, dips, eggs, smoothies, and stir-fries. Or for a bit of added crunch, cut turmeric into thin matchsticks for salads.

As a general rule, 1 tablespoon of freshly grated turmeric is equal to 1 teaspoon of the ground spice.

Store fresh turmeric in an airtight container in the fridge for up to two weeks.

Got GERD? Tap into turmeric's healing powers

No doubt about it. Turmeric will add a glorious shade of gold to your tasty curries and stews. But this aromatic spice's powers don't stop there. Long valued as a traditional medicine, natural compounds in turmeric have been found to slow unwanted hair growth, cleanse wounds, and help neutralize deadly cobra venom.

One of those compounds — a polyphenol called curcumin — acts as a strong antioxidant and anti-inflammatory. Those powers may prove essential in the treatment of gastroesophageal reflux disease (GERD).

One study designed to mimic the effects of stomach acid backwash on people with GERD found that curcumin blocked cytokine activity in esophageal cells. How does that help? Cytokines are powerful proteins known to cause inflammation.

Scientists also looked at how curcumin might help people with Barrett's esophagus — a condition in which GERD causes abnormal cellular changes to the lining of the lower esophagus. Those changes are thought to increase the risk of developing cancer.

The researchers found that a daily dose of 500 milligrams of curcumin over seven days doubled the frequency of apoptosis — that is, the rate at which dysfunctional cells die on schedule — in people with Barrett's esophagus.

Why is that good? One of the hallmarks of cancer is the ability of abnormal cells to evade apoptosis, divide without control, and invade surrounding tissue or spread to other parts of the body.

The joys of roughing it — heal your heartburn with a fiber fix

Ever eat a pine tree? Seems like you couldn't turn on the TV in the early 1970s without running across Grape-Nuts spokesman Euell Gibbons asking that very question. Gibbons, though, was more than a pop culture sensation. He was an avid outdoorsman who knew a thing or two about eating right. And he was on the mark with Grape-Nuts. Just half a cup of the crunchy cereal packs a hefty 7 grams of fiber.

You probably know that fiber helps keep your digestive tract running smoothly. It turns out that it also may provide relief from heartburn and bitter acid backwash.

Fiber gives reflux a run for the money. A study of 36,539 Norwegians found that those who ate bread with a low fiber content were roughly twice as likely to experience acid reflux symptoms than people who ate high-fiber bread. The researchers weren't exactly sure why fiber seems to protect against acid reflux.

However, they think it might be related to fiber's ability to hunt down and scoop up nitrites — compounds that are produced naturally when you eat certain foods and are added to others, like processed meat, as a preservative — in your stomach. That, in turn, cuts down on the concentration of nitric oxide in the area where your stomach meets your esophagus.

Why is that important? Because nitric oxide relaxes your lower esophageal sphincter, the gatekeeper responsible for preventing stomach acid from seeping into your gullet.

> Thinking of adding more fiber to your diet? Go slow. Adding too much too quickly can be tough on your digestive system, causing your belly to bloat and cramp. Slowly add a mixture of high-fiber friends like pears, apples, beets, artichokes, split peas, lentils, oats, and popcorn.

Psyllium is stellar at curbing heartburn. Looks like psyllium — the constipation-fighting fiber supplement sold in stores as Metamucil — works double duty when it comes to your health.

That's what Russian researchers discovered after testing the effects of 15 grams of psyllium a day — about 12.5 grams of soluble fiber — on 30 adults accustomed to eating a low-fiber diet. All of the participants had a type of gastroesophageal reflux disease (GERD) that doesn't cause visible injury to the esophagus. They were encouraged to stick to their normal daily activities and not change their eating habits.

After just 10 days, the frequency of their GERD symptoms fell dramatically. The researchers say the results may be due to fiber's nitrite-hunting skills. In addition, they say, some fibers may also neutralize stomach acid.

The crux of reflux — healthy habits to halt the pain

You're not alone if your favorite late night snack — say, leftover pizza or a bowl of chocolate ice cream — suddenly leaves you feeling like an amateur fire eater. Lots of seniors develop acid indigestion from foods that never used to cause trouble.

Common reasons include weight gain, medications, a slowing digestive system, and even missing teeth. Fortunately, you can take simple steps to beat the heat of heartburn.

A Polish study of more than 500 people found several common risk factors among adults with symptoms of gastroesophageal reflux disease (GERD), including pain and fullness in the upper abdomen after eating and a "lump in the throat" feeling.

Not surprisingly, the volunteers with GERD reported a strong link between symptom flare-ups and what they ate. The main culprits? Foods that are fatty, spicy, fried, and sour.

The participants with GERD also tended to consume more citrus fruits and juices, tomatoes, and chocolate than the healthy control group.

Researchers also discovered the following details about the habits of the GERD sufferers.

- They were more likely than the control group to eat one to two meals a day. Researchers say to stick to at least three meals a day, though four to five small ones may be even better for GERD symptoms.

- The participants with GERD tended to skip lunch and gobble up a large meal in the evening. Instead, you should eat regularly throughout the day. Eating a healthy lunch, for example, lowers your chances of overeating at dinner.

- They were prone to drinking peppermint tea. The scientists say the volunteers with GERD may have mistakenly thought the drink would ease symptoms. But research suggests the contrary. Peppermint may encourage acid backwash by relaxing the sphincter muscle between your stomach and esophagus, so you may want to avoid it.

Taking a stand: A simple strategy to slash symptoms

Uh-oh. You stuffed yourself silly at this year's over-the-top Thanksgiving feast. Now the couch is calling. You grab the remote, lie down, and begin to nod off. Seems like a good way to recover your pre-dinner energy, right?

Not if you're prone to heartburn. Lying down makes it easier for stomach acid to seep into your esophagus. In addition, sleeping causes your stomach to empty slowly and produce more acid.

After eating, wait at least three hours before laying down. Stand and walk around to get your gastric juices flowing in the right direction.

These after-meal tips may also lower your chances of developing heartburn.

- Drink a small glass of water and chew gum to neutralize stomach acid.

- Avoid tight-fitting waistbands that squeeze your belly.

- Don't drink carbonated liquids. Bloating can cause stomach acid to rise.

High blood pressure

4 easy eats that steady your BP

True or false? These symptoms are all signs of high blood pressure — headaches, blurry vision, and dizziness. The answer? Sort of true, and kind of false. Because some people do have those symptoms, but most people have no signs at all. The only way to know for sure if you have high blood pressure, also known as hypertension, is to let your numbers do the talking.

As your heart pumps blood, sending energy, oxygen, and nutrients all through your body, the blood pushes against the sides of your arteries. The strength of this "pushing" is what's measured when you take your blood pressure.

- The top number — called systolic pressure — represents the pressure in your blood vessels as your heart beats.

- The bottom number, diastolic pressure, is measured when your heart rests between beats.

Experts say to shoot for a reading below 120/80 millimeters of mercury (mmHg). So how high is too high? Recently, the American Heart Association and the American College of Cardiology lowered the definition of high blood pressure from 140/90 mmHg to 130/80 mmHg. That means nearly half of American adults now fall into the high blood pressure category.

Lifestyle choices could be making it worse. Smoking, stress, and

Eat

Apples	Apricots
Beetroot juice	Blueberries
Low-fat dairy	Spinach
Walnuts	Watermelon
Pomegranate juice	

Avoid

Salt

Sugar

Grilled meats

Processed meat like bacon or hot dogs

excess body fat can cause your blood pressure to get too high, damaging your arteries. And this can lead to some life-altering problems like stroke, vision loss, heart attack, kidney disease — even dementia.

Don't worry. You can eat your way to healthier blood pressure. It's simple. Just add a few of these delicious foods to your menu every day.

> And while you're at it, top off your lunch hour with watermelon. This juicy fruit contains L-citrulline, an amino acid that helps your body make the same nitric oxide known to help lower your BP.

Go a little nutty at breakfast. In a recent study of more than 2,000 healthy adults, those with the most omega-3 fatty acids in their blood also had the lowest blood pressure readings.

Interesting, perhaps, but what does that mean for you? Researchers think omega-3 fatty acids may help the walls of your blood vessels relax and widen, improving blood flow and helping your blood pressure go down. Got your attention now, right?

To add heart-healthy omega-3 to your diet, just toss some delicious English walnuts on your morning oatmeal. A 1-ounce serving — about 1/4 cup — provides 2,565 milligrams (mg) of omega-3.

Nuts not your thing? Perk up your breakfast smoothies with a tablespoon of whole flaxseed, which contains 2,338 mg of omega-3. Or taste test a tablespoon of flaxseed oil, which offers a whopping 7,196 mg.

Snack time calls for berries. If you're at all concerned about high blood pressure, eat delicious blueberries. These little powerhouses are packed with pigments called anthocyanins, antioxidants that may work their magic by making your blood vessels more elastic.

Researchers discovered this after looking at data on more than 156,000 participants from the Nurses' Health Study (NHS) I, NHS II, and Health Professionals Follow-up Study. They found that people who ate the most anthocyanins from blueberries and strawberries had an 8% drop in their risk for high blood pressure, compared to those who ate the lowest amounts.

And according to experts at Harvard Medical School, it only takes 1 1/2 cups per week — of either berry — to enjoy heart benefits.

Lunch on leafy greens. Found in spinach, kale, cabbage, and other leafy greens, nitrates lower your blood pressure by producing nitric oxide, a gas that helps your blood vessels relax and makes your arteries more flexible. "We were surprised by how little nitrate was needed to see such a large effect," says Amrita Ahluwalia, lead author of a study published in the journal *Hypertension*. The research shows that the amount of nitrates found in a large bowl of lettuce could lower your blood pressure about 11 points.

Add apricots to the menu for a super supper. You probably know eating less salt goes hand in hand with lower blood pressure. But did you know you need potassium, too? Potassium partners with your kidneys to get rid of extra sodium. And it relaxes your blood vessel walls which lowers your blood pressure, too.

Dr. Alicia McDonough, author of a recent review on the BP-lowering effects of potassium, says reducing your sodium intake is a great place to start, but you can do more. "Evidence suggests that increasing dietary potassium may have an equally important effect on hypertension."

And it's an easy fix. Just 1 cup of dried apricots provides more than 40% of your daily requirement of potassium. Other lip-smacking ideas — add a cup of cooked lentils or a hearty baked potato to your evening meal.

You forgot your Amazon password — again. But memory loss is just a part of getting old, right? Consider this. The culprit could be high blood pressure (HBP). One study found HBP could prematurely age your brain by seven years. And even slightly elevated pressure raises your dementia risk. To maintain a razor-sharp brain, keep that blood pressure right on the numbers.

Salt shakedown: New health dangers revealed

It adds zing to foods. It cures meat and preserves vegetables. In moderation, it regulates your heartbeat and your body's balance of fluids. But get too much salt and you're in for a world of problems. In fact, researchers say eating too much salt may lead to well over 1 million deaths worldwide every year.

- Higher salt intake means higher blood pressure. That's because salt causes your body to retain water, increasing the amount of blood in your arteries. It also causes small arteries to constrict, making it harder for blood to squeeze through.

- The resulting high blood pressure increases your risk for heart attack and stroke.

Scientists came to these conclusions after gathering information from over 60 countries. But the Institute of Medicine says more research needs to be done to see if less salt in your diet lowers your risk of heart disease.

You don't want to cut salt out completely. Your body needs sodium to contract muscles, send and receive nerve signals, and regulate fluids and electrolytes. But how much, exactly?

Remember, Dietary Reference Intakes, or DRIs, include Recommended Dietary Allowances (RDAs) and Adequate Intakes (AIs). RDA levels tell you how much of a nutrient most healthy people of a particular age group and gender should get each day. AIs are set when scientists have too little data to establish an RDA value.

Since no Recommended Dietary Allowance has been established for sodium, a committee of nutrition experts from the Food and Nutrition Board set an AI instead. So the amount you should have, based on estimates of the salt intake by groups of healthy people, is 1,300 milligrams a day for ages 51 to 70, and 1,200 milligrams a day for people over age 70.

The kicker is you really only need a smidgeon of sodium for your body to work properly. A mere 500 milligrams per day — that's less than 1/4 teaspoon of salt — should do the trick. Experts say if you have diabetes, high blood pressure, chronic kidney disease, are over age 51, or African American you should definitely cut back.

So watch your blood pressure and keep an eye on your salt intake. Your heart will welcome the much-needed break.

Steer clear of sodium hiding in your favorite foods

You're serious about bringing down your blood pressure. But how can you lower your numbers if you don't know where the sodium is lurking? It's like playing a game of hide-and-seek — with some pretty serious health consequences.

Watch out for these popular foods that contain more sodium than you might think.

Food	Serving size	Amount of sodium
frozen buttermilk pancakes	3 pancakes	815 mg
jarred spaghetti sauce	1/2 cup	525 mg
canned chicken noodle soup	1 cup	474 mg
low-fat cottage cheese	1/2 cup	459 mg
canned mushrooms	1/2 cup	331 mg
kosher dill pickles	1 spear	306 mg
unfrosted chocolate cake	1 slice	299 mg
light Italian salad dressing	2 tbsp	228 mg
rye bread	1 slice	211 mg
ketchup	1 tbsp	167 mg

Lower the salt, raise the flavor with these tasty tips

Why not skip the salt and use herbs instead to deliciously season your food? Try fresh basil, rosemary, mint, or oregano for starters. Or how about adding black pepper, cinnamon, or turmeric? You might like to try grinding dried spices yourself for added freshness.

And don't be afraid to use some good-for-you fats in your cooking, too. Healthy oils like olive, soybean, and canola can add a rich flavor to meals — without extra sodium. You can even get a little fancy with flavored oils like truffle oil or garlic-infused oils.

But sometimes what your food really needs is just a little acid, not salt. Try some lemon juice or apple cider vinegar to brighten up your dish. Some citrus zest can work miracles — and there's no extra salt to worry about.

9 ways to cut out sneaky salt

Salt seems to be hiding everywhere, doesn't it? Trying to rid your diet of extra sodium may seem like an assignment for the Mission Impossible crew. But you don't have to call Martin Landau, Barbara Bain — or even Tom Cruise — for help. Here are some easy ways you can cut back on the amount of salt you get every day. No secret agents needed.

Eat fewer processed foods. Just laying off the saltshaker won't solve the problem of too much sodium. A whopping 77% of the salt you eat each day comes from prepackaged foods and restaurant meals, not from the salt on your own table. Manufacturers add salt during processing to punch up flavor and lengthen a food's shelf life. Cut back on canned vegetables and soups, broths, frozen dinners, instant rice and pasta mixes, cheeses, salad dressings, snack foods, and fast foods. Switch to eating more fresh fruits and vegetables, and you'll automatically eat less salt.

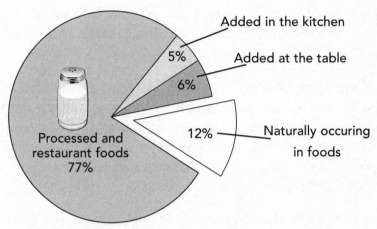

You control over 88% of the salt in your diet.

Read labels for sodium content and serving size. Breads and pastries that taste sweet, not salty, are actually some of the biggest contributors to dietary sodium. Read every food's label to avoid unpleasant surprises. For instance, you may think coffee is bad for your blood pressure, but drinking sodas may be worse. In fact, having too much of this everyday drink could be what's raising your blood pressure, since a single 12-ounce can contains about 50 milligrams (mg) of sodium.

The Nutrition Facts panel tells you how many milligrams of sodium are in a single serving of food. Check the serving size against how much you plan to eat in one sitting.

Buy fresh or frozen fish, poultry, and meat. These tend to have less salt than their canned and processed counterparts. Whenever possible, avoid cold cuts, bacon, and ham. Even those oh-so-convenient rotisserie chickens in your grocery store are pre-treated with salt.

Go easy on the condiments. A lot of salt in your diet comes from sauces, like ketchup, mustard, steak and soy sauce, and extras like pickles. Would you believe a large dill pickle contains over 1,000 mg of salt? Treat even low-sodium versions of soy and teriyaki sauces like salt, and use them sparingly.

Prepare it yourself. Whenever possible, cut back on restaurant meals. Make your own dishes from scratch and it will be harder for salt to sneak up on you.

Be stingy when cooking. Try using half the salt called for in any recipe. Or cut it out completely. You can always add a bit at the table. Just don't salt your food automatically, like many people do. At least taste it first, and if you feel it needs a little something, try pepper, onion or garlic powder, or a salt-free commercial product, like Mrs. Dash.

Rinse canned foods. You can cut the sodium in canned vegetables up to 40% just by rinsing them with water before you eat them.

Raid your medicine cabinet. Many over-the-counter and prescription drugs — from antacids and laxatives to pain relievers and cold medicines — contain sodium, too. Read package labels on OTCs and ask your pharmacist to check the inserts that come with prescription drugs.

Switch to a lifesaving substitute. Consider swapping your regular salt for a potassium-enriched salt substitute made with half potassium chloride and half sodium chloride. You'll swing a one-two punch at heart disease by cutting sodium and boosting your potassium intake. Research shows that using this seasoning could reduce deaths from heart disease, diabetes, high blood pressure, and stroke by 40%.

Beware, potassium can be harmful in large amounts, especially if you have kidney disease or take certain medications, including ACE inhibitors and potassium-sparing diuretics such as spironolactone. Talk to your doctor before trying potassium salt substitutes if you fit this description.

3 mighty minerals KO HBP

Gold, silver, and platinum. Among the world's most precious — and priciest — minerals. But when it comes to your good health, they can't hold a candle to the powerhouse minerals your body needs to keep high blood pressure (HBP) at bay.

This amazing "un-salt" keeps BP good and low. What's the "un-salt," you may ask? Why potassium, of course. It works by helping your body get rid of the excess sodium that can raise your blood pressure. Scientists discovered that people with high blood pressure who increased their potassium intake ended up lowering their systolic blood pressure — the top number — by almost 3 1/2 points and dropped their diastolic pressure — the bottom number — by almost 2 points.

To hike up your potassium closer to the daily reference intake (DRI) of 4,700 milligrams, try adding these three tasty snack foods to your meal plan. Start with a banana at breakfast for 422 milligrams (mg) of potassium. Add 1/2 cup of apricots to your lunch for an additional 755 mg. Then enjoy a sweet 1/2 cup of raisins, and you'll add on 598 mg more.

Crush HBP with dairy foods. Seems like good news for you ice cream lovers. A Harvard study confirms that you should eat more low-fat dairy products in order to bring down your blood pressure. Turns out calcium is the magic mineral that helps your blood vessels tighten and relax when they need to, helping to keep your blood pressure steady.

But don't head off for a chocolate shake just yet. The healthiest source of this must-have mineral is low-fat dairy. Enjoy foods like low-fat yogurt or skim milk. Maybe even sneak in a cup of frozen yogurt now and then. Just make sure it's low-fat.

Low zinc can mean high pressure. The mineral zinc has important jobs to do in your body, like helping with nerve and immune function. But researchers have now found a connection between low zinc levels and high blood pressure.

A recent study of more than 140 people showed those with pre-hypertension — blood pressure readings of 120 to 139 mmHg over 80 to 89 mmHg — had significantly lower zinc levels than those with normal blood pressure. The researchers suggest low zinc can go hand in hand with prehypertension, a warning sign that HBP may be in your future.

How does it work? Experts think low zinc levels could change the way kidneys handle sodium, leading to higher blood pressure.

So when it comes to a healthy diet for lowering HBP, think zinc. Remember the old slogan for Wheaties — The Breakfast of Champions? Well, it's true. Just 3/4 cup of good ol' Wheaties will supply you with almost 7 mg of zinc. And with a DRI of 8 to 11 mg, just one bowl puts you well on your way to healthier blood pressure.

Drop your pressure with 2 delicious meal plans

You cruise by that fast-food joint and catch a tantalizing whiff of beef sizzling on the grill. The siren call for burger-loving humans. So what should you do? Pull into the drive-thru and indulge in a quarter-pound patty? Nope. Not if you're serious about dropping those blood pressure numbers.

Researchers have discovered that eating red meat, both the processed — think hot dogs or bacon — and the unprocessed kind — like your favorite burger — can raise your blood pressure and your cholesterol. Not only can high cholesterol up your risk for stroke, heart attack, and heart disease, but it can also cause the buildup of plaque on the walls of your blood vessels. And that plaque buildup can block your arteries and lead to high blood pressure.

Meir Stampfer, professor of epidemiology and nutrition at Harvard T.H. Chan School of Public Health, suggests swapping your red meat meals for plant proteins to lower your risk of heart disease. "If you replace burgers with cookies or fries," he says, "you don't get healthier. But if you replace red meat with healthy plant protein sources, like nuts and beans, you get a health benefit." Like lower blood pressure.

These two heart-healthy food plans may even help you forget about that tasty burger.

- **Dietary Approaches to Stop Hypertension (DASH) diet.** Since 1997, researchers have known that a diet rich in fruits, vegetables, and low-fat dairy, with reduced saturated and total fat can lower your blood pressure. Swap out your red meat, sweet treats, and sugary drinks for whole grains, poultry, fish, and nuts, and you could see your systolic pressure drop by almost 6 points in as little as eight weeks.

- **Mediterranean diet.** After a study of more than 1,100 men and women between the ages of 65 and 79, experts found that the Mediterranean diet plan lowered systolic blood pressure in men by around 9 points. The diet was a winner with women, too, who noted an improvement in arterial stiffness — the loss of elasticity and flexibility in arteries that leads to high blood pressure. And if you're truly a carnivore at heart, you can even enjoy an occasional serving of meat — once a week or less — but try to stick mostly to fish or seafood. Enjoy vegetables, fruits, beans, nuts, and whole grains, and don't forget small daily servings of yogurt or soft cheeses like feta.

Cut back on grilling for better blood flow

Grill masters take note. Scientists at an American Heart Association conference reported some sizzling new research.

- Folks who ate grilled, broiled, or roasted meat more than 15 times a month had a 17% greater risk of developing high blood pressure than those who ate similarly prepared meat less than four times a month.

- And chowing down on well-done meats rather than rarer meats was linked to a 15% greater risk for high blood pressure.

Researchers believe the reason has to do with the way your body reacts to the chemicals in grilled fare.

"It may help reduce the risk of high blood pressure if you don't eat these foods cooked well done and avoid the use of open-flame and high-temperature cooking methods including grilling, barbecuing, and broiling," says lead author Gang Liu, a nutrition researcher at Harvard School of Public Health.

Fruit of the bloom: 2 superfruits stem the tide of HBP

The apple and the pomegranate have more in common than you might think. For starters, both fruits have been around for thousands of years. And both have survived the stigma of being stuck with the wicked nickname "forbidden fruit." Just try living that one down.

But these fruits have something else in common that's quite unexpected. When it comes to high blood pressure, they both get right to the root of the problem.

Get some skin in the game to lower your blood pressure.
Apple skin, that is. This crunchy way to lower your blood pressure is delicious and cheap — and you don't even need a doctor's prescription to get started.

Apples contain quercetin, a special chemical found in a rainbow of fruits and vegetables. Researchers say quercetin helps lower your blood pressure by encouraging your body to rid itself of excess fluids and salt. This helps reduce the pressure in your arteries.

> Some people think sea salt is better for them, because it's less processed. But sea salt and table salt have the same amount of sodium, so don't think you're eating healthier because you've switched over. Most salt comes from the sea anyway. Focus on the amount of salt you're getting, not the source.

But experts know most of the apple's quercetin is in its skin, so don't send that color-packed peel down the garbage disposal. Instead, enjoy every single bite to keep your blood pressure in check.

Keep your arteries young with the "grainy apple." Surprise, that's another term for the pomegranate. And another surprise, just a single cup of refreshing pomegranate juice every day is enough to keep cholesterol from turning into artery-clogging plaque. Scientists think the antioxidants in pomegranate juice do the work for you by preventing hardening of the arteries and reducing blood vessel damage. These powerful antioxidants may even reverse the damage that's already been done.

Pomegranate juice reduces the effects of stress on your blood vessels by juicing up the production of nitric oxide, a chemical that helps keep your arteries wide open and your blood flowing like it should.

And you can just leave your other juices in the fridge. One group of volunteers agreed to a daily serving of pomegranate. At the end of the study, researchers discovered the volunteers had lower blood pressure and less thickening of the artery walls.

So savor the flavor of pomegranate juice and apples, a tasty power pair from ancient times. They're ready and waiting to battle your high blood pressure.

To lower high pressure, just beet it

Your mom was right — eat your beets. This bright red super-food from your childhood dinner table has the power to lower your blood pressure today. And now you can trade in your fork for a straw.

Researchers discovered that folks who drank 1 cup of beet-root juice daily lowered their systolic BP by more than 11 points and their diastolic BP by almost 10 points. And the effects were still there after 24 hours. Turns out beetroot juice contains nitrates that change to nitric oxide (NO) in your body. This chemical compound is released by cells in your blood vessels, causing them to widen and relax.

Making your own juice is easy peasy. Just chop your beets and toss them in your blender with a little water. Add your favorite greens or fruit, if desired. Blend until the mixture has a juice-like consistency. Pour through a fine-mesh strainer into your glass and enjoy.

Stop the pop to help your heart

You know sodium can raise your blood pressure and damage your blood vessels. But your HBP may not be just salt's fault. Instead, it could be caused by that icy cold bottle of sugary soda in the fridge.

Want to lower your blood pressure? Take a look at this hard news about soft drinks.

Researchers tracked 810 adults, ages 25 to 79, who had participated in an 18-month study focused on weight loss, exercise, and a healthy diet as a way to control blood pressure.

- At the beginning of the study, participants drank just under one serving of a sugar-sweetened beverage each day. The sugary drinks included regular soft drinks, fruit drinks, lemonade, and fruit punch. Diet drinks were not counted.

- At the end of the study, the group's sugary drink consumption averaged half a serving per day.

And the impact on blood pressure? Researchers found a statistically significant drop.

Experts think one way the sugar-sweetened drinks increase BP is by raising the level of uric acid — a waste product of digestion and the culprit behind gout.

Too much uric acid can lower the amount of nitric oxide your body has available to keep your blood vessels wide open, your blood flowing freely, and your blood pressure down.

There's just no sugarcoating this bottom line. "Our findings suggest that reducing sugar-sweetened beverages and sugar consumption may be an important dietary strategy to lower blood pressure and further reduce other blood pressure-related diseases," says Liwei Chen, M.D., Ph.D., assistant professor at Louisiana State University Health Science Center School of Public Health. Good advice for your heart.

Cocoa gets high-fives for fighting ticker troubles

Chocolate and hearts go hand-in-hand, and not just on Valentine's Day. A little chocolate every day will keep your heart beating for years to come.

Fabulous flavanols battle heart disease. That's what two separate studies proved when they tested cocoa drinks on healthy adults up to 80 years old. Participants drank beverages with or without cocoa flavanols twice a day for either two or four weeks.

At the end of both studies, those who drank the real cocoa showed one or more of these benefits.

• lower blood pressure

• better blood flow

• lower bad LDL cholesterol and higher good HDL cholesterol

• flexible blood vessels

• lower risk of heart disease

According to researcher Malte Kelm, cardiology professor at University Hospital Düsseldorf, cocoa can have long-term benefits for your heart.

"Our results indicate that dietary flavanol intake reduces the 10-year risk of being diagnosed with CVD (cardiovascular disease) by 22% and the 10-year risk of suffering a heart attack by 31%," he says.

Cocoa tops the charts for heart benefits. Based on previous studies, scientists know cocoa flavanols help people who are at high risk or who already have heart disease. These two studies focused on low-risk adults with no signs of heart problems. As you can see, the results show flavanols benefit healthy adults, too.

So no matter what group you fall into — healthy, at-risk, or diagnosed with heart disease — you can drink cocoa to your heart's content.

But before you raid the pantry for your favorite hot cocoa mix, listen up. It's the natural, unsweetened powder that's good for you, not the sugary stuff you top with marshmallows and whipped cream on cold, wintry nights.

Unsweetened cocoa powder contains the highest number of flavanols and won't add inches to your waist. One tablespoon has only 12 calories. Other chocolate products have fewer flavanols because of the way they're processed.

Ranked from highest to lowest in flavanols are cocoa powder, baking chocolate, dark chocolate or baking chips, milk chocolate, and chocolate syrup. Notice the pattern? The sweeter the chocolate, the fewer nutrients it contains.

More cocoa? Yes, please! Finding ways to add unsweetened cocoa to your diet is the best way to boost your flavanol intake. These ideas will get you started.

- Mix frozen banana slices and cocoa powder in a blender until smooth for a creamy treat.

- Make granola bars with rolled oats, your favorite nut butter, a little honey or agave syrup, chopped nuts or seeds, and a dusting of cocoa powder.

- Sprinkle over popcorn while you catch up on your favorite flicks.

- Add a tablespoon to a pot of beef stew or chili.

Inflammatory bowel disease

Heal your gut from the inside out

Can you guess what John F. Kennedy and Dwight D. Eisenhower had in common? Aside from the fact that both men were president of the United States, they also suffered from inflammatory bowel disease (IBD).

This term refers to two conditions — Crohn's disease (CD) and ulcerative colitis (UC) — that cause parts of your digestive tract to become inflamed. Both lead to abdominal pain, weight loss, fatigue, and diarrhea.

Because these chronic illnesses affect your gut, scientists think the treatment might be there, too. So researchers started looking for answers in the microbiome. That's the name for the trillions of microorganisms that live not only in your digestive system but throughout your body, as well.

Don't worry — most of these bacteria, fungi, parasites, and viruses help you break down food, absorb nutrients, and fight off disease. But what experts have discovered is that many people suffering from IBD also have an unhealthy microbiome, one where the harmful bacteria outweigh the good.

And that's why you want to make sure yours is in tiptop shape. First step — eat foods loaded with helpful bacteria, called probiotics.

This fermented food will get your gut back on track. You might think of yogurt as just a healthy snack or quick breakfast.

Eat	
Probiotic yogurt	Fatty fish
Olive oil	Chicory root
Whole grains	Mangoes
Green tea	Walnuts

Avoid	
Butter	Alcohol
Gluten	Meat

But researchers recently published a study that suggests this treat could hold the key to fighting IBD flare-ups.

They split over 200 people with IBD into two groups. Half were asked to eat a probiotic yogurt every day, and the other half were given a yogurt substitute.

At the end of eight weeks, those in the probiotic yogurt group experienced less nausea, vomiting, bloating, and diarrhea. Experts say that's because the probiotics increased the amount of good bacteria in their guts.

If you want to try this for yourself, eat about a cup of yogurt containing live cultures of *Lactobacillus acidophilus LA5* and *Bifidobacterium BB12* every day.

Look outside the dairy aisle. Yogurt isn't the only way to get probiotics. Supplements containing live cultures may give you protection from IBD symptoms, too. In fact, you might actually prefer pills and capsules to yogurt, particularly if you're lactose intolerant. In addition, these products can make it easy to find and take specific strains of bacteria.

When you're shopping for supplements, keep these tips in mind.

- Tally up the CFUs. The colony forming units, or CFUs, are a measure of a probiotic's strength. For instance, in the IBD study, those eating probiotic yogurt got about 26,500 CFUs a day.

- Check the date. The bacteria are only guaranteed to be active as long as the supplement isn't past the use-by date.

- Make sure the strain matches your needs. Read the fine print to see if you're buying the right one.

- Scan the label for storage instructions. Some probiotics need to be stashed in the fridge instead of the medicine cabinet. Make sure the store you're buying from follows the directions, and do the same when you get home.

Surprising way to fuel your microbiome

So your microbiome is now teeming with the perfect mix of good bacteria. But wait, you can't stop there.

Imagine trying to run a mile after chowing down on a greasy hamburger and fries, with a chocolate milkshake chaser. That's not the right fuel for a healthy body. The same is true for your microbiome. Your gut bacteria need the right food to do their job.

What exactly should you feed your gut, you may ask? Prebiotics. Experts say the helpful bacteria in your body thrive on this particular group of nutrients, which includes specific fiber, starches, and sugars you can't otherwise digest. One prebiotic in particular, inulin, has successfully treated ulcerative colitis.

Inulin is found naturally in asparagus, onions, and garlic, but you can always take a supplement. Most commercial products are made from chicory root, an extremely rich source of inulin.

Triple threat — 3 tasty diets keep IBD at bay

Sugary snacks or spicy foods can be an IBD sufferer's worst nightmare. On the other hand, the right foods are your tummy's dream come true. Experts say these three diets fit the bill.

The Mediterranean diet. Several studies show this eating plan can reduce inflammation in the guts of people with IBD, and increase the amount of healthy bacteria in their microbiomes.

It emphasizes healthy fats, fish, legumes, vegetables, and whole grains. And that means you're getting a heaping helping of good-for-you omega-3 fatty acids and fiber, but few omega-6 fatty acids and saturated fats. These unhealthy fats — which include butter and vegetable oil — are known to cause inflammation in high doses. Plus, they have been strongly linked with an increased risk of developing ulcerative colitis (UC) and Crohn's disease (CD).

So how can you follow this diet?

- Go all in on fatty fish. Salmon, tuna, sardines, or mackerel should be a staple on your dinner table. Try to eat them at least twice a week.

- Opt for olive oil. This healthy fat is a great alternative to butter in your cooking.

- Fill up on plants. Try to get seven to 10 servings of fruit and veggies every day.

A plant-based diet. Japanese researchers found that cutting back on animal protein, fat, and sugar, while boosting grains, fruits, and vegetables allows you to battle back against Crohn's symptoms.

A small clinical trial gathered people with Crohn's disease in remission who were at risk of a relapse. They ate a high-fiber, semi-vegetarian diet (SVD) under supervision for up to 82 days, then were discharged from the hospital. After a year, every person who continued with the SVD maintained their remission. And two years later, 92% of those still showed no signs of the disease.

If you want to try this yourself, researchers suggest your eating plan include at least 32 grams of fiber each day. You can get this much from 2 cups of beans and brown rice, a large apple, and a handful of almonds. Easy and delicious.

And while the diet should be mostly fruits and vegetables, you're still allowed to eat dairy and eggs.

The DASH diet. It seems if you guard your heart, you're also protecting your gut. You may know cutting down on sugar, salt, and fat is great for the old ticker. In fact, those changes are the building blocks of the Dietary Approaches to Stop Hypertension — better known as the DASH diet. But now experts think this heart-healthy meal plan could hold some promise for soothing the symptoms of CD and UC.

The reason? The foods that are great for your heart are also rock stars at fighting inflammation. And that means fewer flare-ups in your gut. To follow the DASH diet, make sure to stick to these rules.

- Cut your salt intake to 2,300 milligrams a day — that's about 1 teaspoon of table salt. If you can get that amount lower, even better.

- Get plenty of whole grains. The recommendation is six to eight servings a day.

- Fill up on fruits and veggies every day. You want at least four or five servings of each.

- Take it easy on the meat. Experts say no more than one 6-ounce serving of lean meat, poultry, or fish a day.

Dodge these common triggers to beat the GI blues

Want to fight back against flare-ups? What you eat matters, but so does what you don't. Cut out these common trigger foods to help your distressed gastrointestinal tract feel better.

- Meat. Experts tracked the diets of over 60,000 people and found that those who eat more animal-based protein are at higher risk for ulcerative colitis.

- Gluten. Studies have shown that people with Crohn's disease are more likely to have trouble digesting this grain protein.

- Alcohol. Drinking regularly can increase your risk of flare-ups. One study reported that 75% of people with IBD saw their symptoms worsen after they drank alcohol.

Talk to your doctor and keep a food journal to track your symptoms. Trigger foods vary from person to person, so it may take some time to find which foods to avoid.

Tummy troubles? Put out the fire with 2 superfoods

You might make a beeline for leafy greens and whole grains when you're trying to whip up a healthy meal. But you don't want to miss out on some surprising foods that can help you fight IBD. In fact, these two treats could be the inflammation fighters your diet is missing.

Munch on mangoes to soothe inflammation. In a small study, researchers from the Texas A&M University Department of Nutrition and Food Science asked people with IBD to add mangoes to their diet.

The participants started small and, for eight weeks, slowly increased the amount they ate, to avoid shocking their systems with too much of this fiber-rich fruit at once. By the end of the study, they were up to 200 to 400 grams each day — the equivalent of one to two whole mangoes.

Researchers reported that eating mangoes boosted the levels of friendly bacteria in people's microbiomes, and reduced blood levels of endotoxin, a chemical in your body that signals inflammation.

The reason? Experts credit a specific polyphenol, gallotannins, in mangoes. These natural compounds are easily broken down and absorbed by your intestines. And in turn, your body is better equipped to quench inflammation.

Brew up some powerful protection with green tea. Thousands of years ago, tea was thought to be one of the most potent known medicines. Today, modern researchers are once again exploring tea's healing properties. They found evidence to suggest the polyphenols in green tea can help lower your risk of cancer, Alzheimer's, and other chronic diseases. Researchers even think this delicious beverage can thwart IBD.

Animal studies show promising results. A recent paper published in the journal *Nutrients* suggests green tea compounds can fight inflammation and relieve symptoms in IBD sufferers.

Experts think the most powerful polyphenol in tea is epigallocatechin gallate (EGCG). This natural chemical breaks down as tea gets older, so aged teas — like black or oolong — have less of it.

Before you bring out the kettle, you should know that cold steeping tea may be even healthier. That's because brewing in boiling water will destroy some of tea's natural antioxidants.

Get crackin' — squirrel away walnuts for freshness

Eating 20 to 25 walnuts a day could help you ward off ulcerative colitis symptoms says a new study led by Daniel Rosenberg of the University of Connecticut Health's Center for Molecular Oncology.

But don't stick that bag of pre-shelled walnuts in your pantry. They are loaded with oil and will go bad quickly. So how can you make sure your walnuts don't spoil before you get a chance to eat them?

- Use your fridge. Store them in an airtight container, and they'll last up to three months in the refrigerator. Just keep them far away from strong-smelling foods — like onions — or your walnuts might pick up odd flavors and odors.

- Freeze them. Keeping your walnuts on ice will help them last for up to a year.

You can tell your walnuts are rancid if they are shriveled or smell like paint thinner. Toss 'em out.

Insomnia

Better rest by the bite: 3 foods for a sweet slumber

The sheep were in the meadow. The cow was in the corn. But where was Little Boy Blue and his trusty horn? Sacked out under the haystack, of course. Seems like Blue fell fast asleep without even batting an eye. So why can't you?

Could be lots of reasons. Health conditions like sleep apnea and arthritis, as well as medications to treat high blood pressure and depression, can make it tough to nod off. In addition, worry and stress can keep you tossing and turning all night.

Fortunately, the following fruits contain compounds that are likely to help you fall — and stay — asleep. Read on for a more restful night.

For a good night's sleep, tart cherries are tops. Pass up the sleeping pills and snack on a handful of these tasty, ruby-red treats or savor a glass of tart cherry juice instead. In a recent study, two small groups of seniors who suffered from insomnia were asked to drink 8 ounces of either Montmorency tart cherry juice or a placebo. Folks drank their assigned liquid in the morning and one to two hours before bedtime. After two weeks, researchers found that those who drank the tart cherry juice increased their sleep time by 84 minutes.

What's the secret? It may be that tart cherries are chock-full of melatonin, a hormone that signals

Eat

Tart cherries	Kiwis
Bananas	Raspberries
Almonds	Walnuts
Mustard seed	Honey
Chamomile tea	Quinoa

Avoid

High-glycemic foods like soda and white rice

your body when it's time to sleep. This new research also says the insomnia-fighting power could be the work of a polyphenol called procyanidin B-2.

Slice into kiwi fruit to fall asleep quicker. This small, slightly fuzzy fruit sure packs a lot of sleep-supporting nutrition. A study of 24 adults with difficulty falling or staying asleep found that eating two kiwis an hour before bed greatly improved sleep quality and quantity.

After four weeks of eating the fruit, the total time the volunteers spent sleeping increased 13%. Plus the amount of time it took them to fall asleep dropped 35%. They also woke up less often during the night.

The researchers say the kiwi's high concentrations of antioxidants, serotonin, and folate may be responsible for the dramatic improvements in sleep.

Bring on bananas for a more restful night. Lots of people turn to bananas as their go-to source of potassium, a mineral that's vital to muscle, heart, and kidney function.

But a large banana is also packed with magnesium — about 11% of the daily recommended amount for senior women — which appears to help your body sleep.

A small Iranian study found that seniors who took 500 grams of magnesium supplements daily over eight weeks saw improvements in their insomnia symptoms. They also had significant increases in their levels of melatonin.

It makes sense, considering people who don't get enough magnesium often don't sleep well. Scientists believe magnesium supports a good night's rest by maintaining healthy levels of GABA, a neuro-transmitter that helps regulate anxiety and promote sleep.

Drift off to dreamland with this a-peel-ing tea

Been tossing your banana peels in the trash? That's too bad. You could be making a relaxing tea with them.

You'll want to start with a ripe, organic banana peel. Its skin will be thinner and sweeter than that of a green banana, and will also be free of herbicides and pesticides. Be sure to rinse the peel of any dirt. Trim both ends and place the banana skin in a small saucepan. Add 1 1/4 cups of water and bring to a boil. Cover, reduce heat, and let simmer for 10 minutes.

Strain the banana tea into a mug and let it cool slightly. For added sweetness, try drizzling a bit of honey or maple syrup into the brew. You can also spice up your tea with a dash of nutmeg, cinnamon, or turmeric.

Sip these teas to catch some ZZZs

"If you are cold, tea will warm you; if you are too heated, it will cool you; if you are depressed, it will cheer you; if you are excited, it will calm you." As you can see, William Gladstone, a 19th-century British statesman, was a fan of England's iconic beverage.

But as much as he seemed to enjoy a steaming cuppa, there's something Gladstone forgot to include in his tribute to tea. He could have added, "If you are restless, it will bring you sleep." In other words, a good night's sleep is in the bag. The tea bag, that is — but only if it's one of these herbal, decaffeinated teas.

Cozy up with chamomile to bring on sweet dreams. Scientists believe chamomile tea gets its soothing powers from an antioxidant called apigenin that works in your brain to make you drowsy enough to get the sleep you need. It's even been shown to benefit people with anxiety. Here's what research says.

- In a study of 80 new moms who were having trouble sleeping, researchers found that drinking chamomile tea for two weeks helped relieve symptoms related to sleep problems and depression.

- An eight-week study of 57 volunteers with generalized anxiety disorder found that participants who took chamomile extract showed much greater improvements in their anxiety than those who didn't take the extract.

Valerian gets to the root of the problem. The cure for your sleepless nights might just be valerian, an herb that's been used for centuries to treat nervousness and headaches. And recent studies show valerian helps promote deep sleep, too. Researchers think valerian root may help by increasing levels of the brain neurotransmitter GABA, a chemical messenger that promotes relaxation and sleep.

To make a soothing valerian tea, pour a cup of boiling water over 1 teaspoon of the dried root and steep for five to 10 minutes. For best results, drink your tea two to three hours before bedtime. And be patient. It may take up to a month before you notice results.

Try adding a tablespoon of honey to your tea. The natural sugars prompt your pancreas to release a low amount of insulin. That, in turn, makes it easier for tryptophan — the nap-inducing amino acid in Thanksgiving turkey — to convert into serotonin, a hormone that promotes relaxation and sleep.

Fragrant lavender soothes you to sleep. As far back as ancient Greece, folks knew lavender's soothing fragrance could help relax and settle frayed nerves. And who better to test the calming effects of lavender than that same group of sleep-deprived new moms? After drinking a cup of lavender tea every day for two weeks, the women reported less tiredness and depression.

And for some people, just breathing in the scent of lavender did the trick. One study found that women between the ages of 45 and 55 who received 20 minutes of lavender aromatherapy twice per week for 12 weeks reported a significant improvement in their sleep quality.

Hungry for sleep? Try melatonin-rich foods

Did you know that your body's production of melatonin drops with age? It may be why seniors have higher rates of insomnia than younger folks.

New research suggests just how important melatonin can be when it comes to getting a good night's rest. Scientists did a month-long study of 116 men with delayed sleep-wake phase disorder — a condition that makes it difficult to fall asleep and wake up on time. They found that volunteers who took melatonin supplements an hour before bedtime at least five nights in a row each week fell asleep 34 minutes earlier than those taking a placebo.

Fortunately, you don't have to turn to supplements to get more melatonin. Orange bell peppers, tomatoes, raspberries, and goji berries stick out as superstars. Almonds, walnuts, and flaxseed also contain lots of melatonin, as do spices like mustard seed and fenugreek.

Not getting enough shut-eye? Be a blood sugar sleuth

More than 1 in 3 seniors regularly turn to some sort of medication — prescription, over-the-counter, or herbal — to doze off at night, according to a University of Michigan poll. But using drugs to fight insomnia carries health risks for adults over age 65, including falls, memory issues, dry mouth, next-day drowsiness, and constipation. After all, older adults are often more sensitive to the effects of drugs than younger people.

A safer way to shed sleeplessness may be found in foods with a low glycemic index (GI). Your body takes longer to break down the carbohydrates in low-GI fare like oatmeal and lentils, which keeps your blood sugar on an even keel.

Scientists at Columbia University wanted to explore the relationship between GI and insomnia, so they followed the eating habits of more than 53,000 senior women over several years. They found that participants whose diet had the highest GI were significantly more likely to have insomnia than volunteers with the lowest dietary GI. They also saw that women whose diet included higher amounts of fiber, vegetables, and fruit were less likely to develop insomnia.

Love rice but hate its high glycemic index (GI)? Instead of short-grain white rice, switch to brown or wild rice. They have more moderate GI scores and a higher nutritional value. You can also experiment with GI-friendly grains like barley, bulgur, quinoa, buckwheat, and millet.

Researchers say more studies are needed to prove that high-GI foods cause insomnia in senior women. But they say quickly digested, refined carbohydrates in high-GI foods like soda and white rice — and the rapid increase in blood sugar they cause — may be the culprit.

"When blood sugar is raised quickly, your body reacts by releasing insulin, and the resulting drop in blood sugar can lead to the release of hormones such as adrenaline and cortisol, which can interfere with sleep," says the study's senior author James Gangwisch, assistant professor at Columbia University Vagelos College of Physicians and Surgeons.

Irritable bowel syndrome

Cook up digestive relief with the low-FODMAP diet

Imagine having to cancel a dinner date because your tight, ballooning belly won't stop rumbling and gurgling. Or avoiding public places because you're afraid you won't have immediate access to a restroom. Scenarios like these happen all too often if you're among the 10% to 15% of American adults with irritable bowel syndrome (IBS).

Get to know the ABCs of IBS. Symptoms can be so distressing that IBS patients in one survey say they would give up, on average, 15 years of their lives in exchange for relief from the chronic cramping, gas, diarrhea, and constipation.

Doctors don't know the causes of IBS, but genetics may play a part. It's also possible that faulty communication between the brain and digestive system causes food to move too slowly or quickly through the large intestine.

Unfortunately, there's no cure. But don't despair. It turns out the food on your plate can make a huge difference when it comes to treating IBS.

Low-FODMAP foods soothe digestive woes. Research suggests that a diet low in carbohydrates known as FODMAPs — short for Fermentable Oligosaccharides, Disaccharides, Monosaccharides, and Polyols — reduces symptoms.

In the largest U.S. study of its kind, research dietitians monitored the progress of 84 IBS patients. About half followed the low-FODMAP

Eat
Yogurt	Oatmeal
Turmeric	Kiwi
Peppermint	

Avoid
Garlic	Onions
Wheat	Fried foods
Sugary drinks	

diet over a month. The other half cut down on known IBS triggers like alcohol and large meals during the same period.

At the end of the study, more than 50% of the patients on the low-FODMAP diet saw a major drop in abdominal pain. That compares with just 20% of the control group.

Those eliminating FODMAPs also reported relief from IBS symptoms like bloating and diarrhea. Not surprisingly, they also experienced greater improvements in their quality of life and anxiety levels than those not following the diet.

On a low-FODMAP diet? You don't have to stop eating bread. While most wheat products are a no-go, sourdough could be an option. The yeast and bacteria in these loaves actually break down the FODMAPs, so you can enjoy a slice of bread without worrying about digestive woes.

Carbs are key to treating symptoms. So why does the eating plan work? Researchers believe some folks have difficulty digesting FODMAPs. That gives carbohydrates extra time to ferment in the gut, creating the perfect environment for bloating and diarrhea.

Considering the low-FODMAP diet? It comes in two parts.

- Elimination phase. Give up FODMAP-rich foods for several weeks. If you're sensitive to FODMAPs, you'll start to feel better pretty quickly.

- Reintroduction phase. Slowly begin eating high-FODMAP foods, one at a time, to identify the ones that cause your IBS symptoms to return.

The following table gives an overview of some high-FODMAP foods you'll have to avoid at first. Be sure to check with your doctor before changing your diet.

FODMAP	Top food sources
Oligosaccharides (fructans, galactans)	wheat, rye, onions, garlic, artichokes, most legumes
Disaccharides (lactose)	milk, yogurt, ice cream, cottage cheese
Monosaccharides (excess fructose)	honey, agave, apples, pears, watermelon
Polyols (sorbitol, mannitol)	stone fruits, mushrooms, cauliflower, sugar-free gum and candy

Get your belly back on track to keep IBS at bay

The ancient Greek physician Hippocrates once said "all disease begins in the gut." There may be some truth to that. Your gut is home to your microbiome, which is made up of trillions of microorganisms that help you digest food, fight illness, and even ward off chronic diseases.

If healthy bacteria don't flourish in your microbiome, you're more likely to have problems with digestion, cramps, bloating, and other symptoms of irritable bowel syndrome. Fortunately, the right foods can help you head off these aches and pains.

Make a few million new friends to protect your gut. Sometimes you need to add helpful bacteria to your microbiome. Why not go straight to the source? Probiotics — live cultures of friendly microbes — are a great way to help your digestive system.

Recently, experts examined 11 studies that proved probiotics can help fend off IBS problems. They concluded that multi-strain supplements, especially those with *Lactobacillus* and *Bifidobacterium*, significantly improved IBS symptoms, including abdominal pain and bloating.

It took about two months before the effects kicked in, so if you don't notice any improvement at first, give your gut a bit of time to readjust.

You can find probiotics in drinks, yogurts, or supplements at your local store. Make sure you double-check the expiration dates. If these products are past their prime, you won't get all the helpful microbes you need.

> Probiotic products are not entirely risk-free. One study showed that if you suffer from pancreatitis these supplements can actually increase your risk of dying compared to a placebo. If you're not sure whether you should add probiotics to your diet, consult your doctor first.

Find the right foods to pump up your microbiome. If you want to keep your microbiome healthy, you need to feed it the right foods. Prebiotics — fibers the bacteria in your gut need to grow — are critical to taming IBS.

One problem with the low-FODMAP diet is that it takes away these fermentable carbs that provide food for your gut microbiota. This changes the bacterial makeup of your colon, and good microbes like *Bifidobacteria* tend to get crowded out.

Spanish researchers wanted to find out whether certain prebiotics would help IBS symptoms better than a low-FODMAP diet as well as how the prebiotics affected gut microbiota. They pitted a Mediterranean-style diet with a prebiotic supplement against a low-FODMAP diet with a placebo supplement.

- Volunteers were asked to follow these diets for four weeks. Researchers analyzed gut bacteria and gas production before and after the special diet, and two weeks after participants switched back to their normal eating habits.

- While both groups had fewer symptoms, only those who took prebiotics had long-lasting improvements. The scientists believe these results were due to positive changes in their microbiome, most notably an increase in *Bifidobacteria*.

These findings show that if you can tolerate prebiotic-rich foods like onion, garlic, asparagus, bran, and bananas, your gut flora will thank you. Try adding a little at a time to see what your system can handle.

Guard your gut with homemade yogurt

Experts say homemade yogurt is a surprisingly effective way to ward off IBS symptoms. And the best part? It's cheap and easy to make. All you need is 2 tablespoons of store-bought yogurt with live cultures and a half gallon of your favorite milk.

- Bring milk to a boil, then simmer for five to 10 minutes. Stir occasionally so the milk doesn't burn.

- Take the milk off the heat and let it cool until lukewarm. You should be able to comfortably put your finger in the milk for several seconds.

- Add a few tablespoons of milk to your yogurt and whisk thoroughly. Transfer the yogurt mixture back to the pot, and stir gently until well mixed.

- Cover the pot with a lid, wrap it in a towel, and put it in an unheated oven with the light on for four to 18 hours. When the yogurt is thick and tangy, place it in the refrigerator for several hours before eating.

The low-carb food plan you need to try

Some people find welcome relief on a low-FODMAP diet, while others regretfully discover it doesn't help. If you still suffer from bloating, cramps, and other painful symptoms, don't despair. Researchers have come up with a different food plan that may just do the trick.

When you cut FODMAPs from your diet, you deprive yourself of many healthy foods, like blackberries, dairy, and even whole-wheat bread. So researchers decided to test an alternative. The starch-and-sucrose-reduced diet (SSRD) simply asks you to eat fewer carbs and sweets.

In a recent Swedish study, scientists selected people with IBS to either follow the SSRD plan or stick with their normal eating habits. After four weeks, they found that those who avoided starches and sugar not only improved their IBS symptoms, they also had more energy and less muscle pain. So how can you do the same?

- Avoid fruits and veggies that are loaded with starch, like bananas, beans, and potatoes. People in the study used the website *sucroseintolerance.com/choosing-your-foods* as a guide.

- Keep your carbohydrate intake low. You should aim to eat more vegetables, fruits, dairy, eggs, and meat in place of breads and cereals.

- Cut sugary juices and desserts out of your diet. If you crave something sweet, enjoy a handful of crunchy nuts instead.

- Chew your food thoroughly to help your body produce amylase, an enzyme vital to breaking down and digesting starch.

3 smart — and delicious — ways to banish the bloat

You know all too well that a cup of coffee in the morning will only lead to an upset stomach. And munching on a plate of greasy fries is a surefire way to end up bloated, gassy, and in pain.

If you deal with irritable bowel syndrome, you probably spend a lot of time focusing on all the things you shouldn't eat. Wouldn't you love to find some foods that will soothe your colon instead of stirring it up? These tasty choices could be just what you need to tame the IBS beast.

Don't get too 'lax' with your herbal supplements

IBS sufferers might be tempted to turn to over-the-counter laxatives for relief, and that can be dangerous. Overdoing them can cause dehydration, weakness, and other severe medical complications.

You may opt for natural remedies, like senna, thinking they are safer than drugs. But even though this herb is an FDA-approved treatment for constipation, it doesn't mean it won't cause problems.

Senna is fine in small doses, but it can cause side effects similar to over-the-counter meds. And long-term use can lead to heart problems and liver damage. To treat constipation, experts recommend a dosage of around 17 milligrams daily for no more than a few days.

You can find senna in supplements or teas, but talk to your doctor before taking it. This herb can cause dangerous interactions with prescription drugs.

Find the right fiber to subdue the spasms. Some experts think IBS sufferers could banish their symptoms by adding more fiber to their diets. But not just any fiber.

- Both types — soluble and insoluble — help keep your digestive tract in top shape. But experts say that getting too much insoluble fiber — like in wheat bran — could cause bloating and cramps in people with sensitive colons.

- Instead, you should focus more on getting soluble fiber from foods like apples, lentils, and oats. This type of fiber will not ferment quickly, so you'll experience less gas and other uncomfortable symptoms.

Studies say you should aim for 20 to 35 grams of fiber each day. But don't pile it on all it once. If your diet is low on fiber, a big

plate of brown rice and broccoli can make you feel like
a bomb is exploding in your
gut. Instead, add a few grams
to your diet every day until
you hit your goal.

If you still need a bit of extra
help, talk to your doctor
about adding a supplement to
your diet. Research suggests
psyllium fiber is a great way
to help fight IBS.

> Enteric-coated peppermint oil capsules are a boon if you suffer from heartburn or GERD in addition to IBS. By bypassing your stomach, the peppermint won't aggravate those conditions. However, if you take medication to lower stomach acid, make sure you pop your peppermint pill at least two hours beforehand or the coating may break down more quickly.

Tummy trouble? Count on kiwi to calm it down. If your stomach
starts rumbling after a burger and shake, grab a fuzzy brown
kiwifruit for dessert. This exotic treat has a special ingredient that
battles bloating.

Kiwis are loaded with a compound called actinidin. This enzyme,
which only kiwis have, quickly breaks down proteins in red meat,
fish, and dairy. The faster your food is digested, the better you'll feel.

For ongoing relief, make this juicy fruit a regular part of your diet.
Researchers asked a group of people with IBS to either take a
kiwi-based extract loaded with actinidin or a placebo. After three
weeks, the kiwi group had less abdominal pain, gas, and bloating.

Get some year-round relief with this holiday treat. Candy
canes. Peppermint tea. Who knew these Christmastime favorites
could help relieve your irritable bowel? The secret lies in peppermint's volatile oil.

Recently, Dutch researchers gathered 190 people with IBS and
split them into groups. Some were asked to take 182 milligrams
of peppermint oil, while others were given a placebo.

After eight weeks, they found peppermint oil significantly reduced abdominal pain, discomfort, and IBS severity. The researchers also noted that peppermint oil in enteric-coated capsules worked best, because they won't dissolve until they get into your small intestine.

Ax inflammation with this golden spice

Are you in on the turmeric craze? This golden spice, which gives many curries their distinct yellow color, is becoming wildly popular in health and nutrition circles. And for good reason. Experts think it could help fight arthritis, prevent Alzheimer's, and even soothe your IBS symptoms.

According to a recent analysis of multiple studies, curcumin — the compound that gives turmeric its yellow hue — could help ward off the inflammation found in IBS sufferers.

Researchers think its unique power to work as both an antioxidant and anti-inflammatory, plus its ability to regulate gut microbiota, could make it a useful tool in your IBS arsenal.

Exactly how much turmeric you need to eat to get these effects is still unclear. The research is still in its early stages, so keep your ear to the ground for more information in the future.

Kidney stones

Tailor your diet to chip away at stone woes

Doctors in the ancient world blamed kidney stones on unwholesome food, and as early as 600 B.C. they surgically removed stones. Thankfully, this painful condition, known also as nephrolithiasis, only requires an operation these days if other treatments fail.

Stones often form when minerals and salts build up and crystallize in your urine. They often pass on their own. You may not even know you've got stones until symptoms hit — lower back pain, nausea, and vomiting are a few.

All kidney stones are unique, but they fall into a category of either calcium or no-calcium stones, depending on what they're made of. Tailoring your diet to the type of stones you are prone to develop can help you prevent future stones from forming.

Eat and drink to prevent calcium stones. Natural substances called oxalates enter your body in foods like nuts, spinach, potatoes, chocolate, wheat bran, rhubarb, and okra. During digestion, they bind with calcium in your gut, then your body eliminates them through stool.

For example, if you eat a modest portion of spinach — a high-oxalate food — for dinner and drink a tall glass of milk, your calcium and oxalates are more likely to bind in your digestive tract before reaching your kidneys. No harm done.

But if you eat the spinach and skip the hydrating, calcium-rich

Eat

Cheese	Coffee
Collard greens	Tea
Figs	Guava
Lemonade	Salmon
Sardines	Water
Yogurt	Cranberry juice

Avoid

Excess red meat or processed meat

High-oxalate foods such as spinach, rhubarb, chocolate, nuts, and potatoes

dairy, the oxalates may not get bound up completely and could head over to your kidneys. Once there, they can crystallize and form calcium oxalate stones — the most common type of kidney stones.

So contrary to popular myth, you shouldn't cut down on calcium. Experts recommend a daily calcium target of 1,200 milligrams, which you can get by eating foods like cheese, yogurt, sardines, and canned salmon. You may also want to consider limiting oxalates.

Hang a no vacancy sign for no-calcium stones. You'll need a different dietary prevention strategy for other types of stones.

- Uric acid. In 10% of cases urine pH is lower than it should be, encouraging these stones to form. Lower your risk of developing them by eating less acid-producing animal protein and more alkaline-forming foods like pasta, beans, fruits, and vegetables.

- Struvite. These stones form when urine pH is neutral or alkaline, which can happen during an upper urinary tract infection. Make your kidneys as unwelcome to stones as possible by drinking acidic beverages like lemonade, cranberry juice, orange juice, coffee, and tea.

- Cystine. Stones form in only 1% of cases with this genetic condition because of high levels of the amino acid cystine built up in your kidneys. Staying hydrated and making your urine more alkaline is helpful, but you may need a doctor's help to treat and prevent these stones.

Risky business — don't take chances with supplements

An orange sits on your kitchen counter next to a couple of supplements — vitamin C and calcium. Should you reach for the pills? If you're a stone former, you may want to leave them on the counter. Here's why.

Cut the concentrated risk by getting C naturally. Large amounts of vitamin C may increase the amount of oxalates and uric acid in your urine, which could lead to kidney stones. In an analysis of 156,735 women in the Nurses' Health Study I and II and 40,536 men in the Health Professionals Follow-up Study, vitamin C supplements were associated with a higher risk of kidney stones in men, but not women.

The good news? Getting vitamin C from food posed no risk of kidney stones, according to the same study. Fruits like guava and papaya and vegetables like sweet red pepper and broccoli are among the best sources of vitamin C. Aim for 90 milligrams (mg) a day for men and 75 mg a day for women.

The perks of caffeine: Take the stick out of stones with a cup of joe

Caffeinated beverages are often added to the "no-no" list for kidney stone formers because of the oxalates. But new research points to reasons that cup of coffee or tea may actually help prevent calcium stones.

In a review of over 200,000 participants from the Health Professionals Follow-up Study and the Nurses' Health Studies I and II, researchers found that participants who consumed the most caffeine had a 26%, 29%, and 31% lower risk of developing stones in each of the respective studies.

Other studies show that drinking caffeinated coffee, decaffeinated coffee, and tea all seem to lower risk, suggesting other nutrients are at play as well. But caffeine seems to be the ringleader for benefits.

Caffeine helps flush out stone-forming substances and may increase urinary citrate. As a result, calcium oxalate stones have a harder time sticking together.

Consider your calcium source. While calcium can help decrease oxalate absorption, if you're a stone former you should be careful with supplements.

As part of the Women's Health Initiative, a large randomized controlled trial analyzed 36,282 women averaging 62 years of age. Researchers discovered that more kidney stones occurred in women taking calcium with vitamin D supplements compared to those in the placebo group.

Researchers aren't sure why supplements are linked to stone formation. Some suspect the risk may be tied to whether you take supplements with or between meals, which could influence how much calcium is available in your gut to bind with oxalate from food. So if possible, stick to calcium-rich foods like collard greens, figs, and yogurt.

Hard evidence to get more potassium than protein

Sure, protein builds your muscles. But did you know animal protein can increase your chances of developing kidney stones? Here's why you should trim down your meat portion and add more servings of fruits and vegetables to your plate.

Measure your meat to slim down your stone risk. Grab a deck of cards and visualize your meat. Two of those make a 6-ounce portion. That's the max daily recommended amount for a 2,000-calorie DASH-style diet — which encourages more fruits and veggies and less red and processed meats. The eating plan is also linked to a lower risk of kidney stones.

Experts think animal protein bumps up kidney stone risk by promoting an acidic environment and increasing the amount of calcium available to crystalize in your urine. That's why this simple measurement strategy may lower your chances of forming uric acid and calcium stones.

Be kind to your kidneys by piling on potassium. Fruits and veggies are alkaline, so when you add them to your plate, you counterbalance acid from animal proteins. One of the key nutrients responsible for this is potassium, a mineral that also lowers urinary calcium levels, protecting against stone formation.

In a cohort study of 193,676 men and women, researchers found that participants who got more potassium in their diets cut their kidney stone risk by up to 56%. Mushrooms, tomato juice, zucchini, apricots, raisins, and guava are all tasty choices packed with potassium.

Skip the hard sell for soft water and save $1,700

If you're thirsty, you're already dehydrated. And if you're a stone former, it means you're cranking up your chances of forming more stones.

Drinking 8 to 12 cups of fluids like water, lemonade, or coffee throughout the day dilutes your urine and your risk of stone formation. Minerals and electrolytes can't hang out together too long in your kidneys to form stones when they're being washed away regularly.

Randomized controlled trial evidence agrees that drinking more H2O could prevent you from getting new stones. But when it comes to water at home, does it matter what kind?

Many people consider water filtration systems for their home because they are concerned about the effects of hard water. It has more calcium carbonate, which could make your water taste bitter, cause buildup in appliances or pipes, and create challenges for cleaning.

Stone formers may worry they are getting too much calcium in hard water. Or sodium if they add a water softener. Potassium softeners are available to soften water without added sodium, but they can cost up to $1,700.

You could benefit from the minerals found naturally in your tap water. After all, you need calcium to prevent further stones. And studies have found no link between water hardness and kidney stone formation.

In fact, according to a new statement in the *British Journal of Urology International*, many calcium oxalate stone formers may be better off drinking their local tap water without filters.

Put your finger on a pulse for nutrition

Cutting back on meat means paring down your chances of uric acid and calcium oxalate stones. Why not substitute some of your meat with a protein-packed pulse — the legume otherwise known as the lentil?

These powerhouses contain oxalates, but this easy preparation practice can lower those levels considerably. When nutrition experts recently soaked lentils in distilled water at a ratio of 1-to-5 for four hours, then cooked them, they found a significant reduction in total oxalates. Remember to discard your cooking water before serving your lentils.

Just 1 cup of cooked lentils has about 16% of your daily value of potassium and small amounts of calcium and vitamin C.

Lentils are so versatile you can use them as a meat substitute in dishes as diverse as chili, lasagna, soup, burgers, tacos, enchiladas, and shepherd's pie. For many recipes, simply sub in 2 cups of cooked lentils for a pound of ground beef.

Memory loss

Recoup your recall with 3 flavorful fruits

"I have a two-story house and a bad memory, so I'm up and down those stairs all the time. That's my exercise," quips Betty White, a popular celebrity who's well into her 90s. You know just what she means. You get up off the couch and walk into the kitchen to get — something — and suddenly you can't remember why you got up.

While Betty White uses her absentmindedness to get a laugh, there's nothing funny about age-related memory loss. That's why you'll want to dig into more of these yummy — and memory-boosting — fruits.

Grapes upgrade nerve function. It appears a refreshing glass of grape juice may ward off Alzheimer's disease. That's according to a small, three-month study of seniors with memory loss.

Researchers found that volunteers who drank about 2 to 2 1/2 cups of Concord grape juice a day performed better on tests involving list-learning and recall.

The scientists say more studies are needed to figure out how the delicious drink boosted their brainpower. But they say anthocyanins — a type of flavonoid that works as an antioxidant — may reduce inflammation and improve nerve function in your brain.

Blueberries bolster blood flow. You'll want to load up on this beloved "brain berry" to reverse age-related mental decline. In one three-month study, healthy adults age 65 and older were separated into two groups. One group drank a cup of juice made

Eat	
Tart cherry juice	Blueberries
Cocoa	Coffee
Sardines	Turmeric
Collard greens	Mushrooms
Sweet potatoes	Walnuts

Avoid	
Fried foods	Butter
Red meat	Cheese

with 2 tablespoons of blueberry concentrate mixed with water. The other group was served a look-alike placebo.

And guess what? Researchers saw more activity in areas of the brain associated with memory in the blueberry drinkers compared to the placebo group. They think blueberries help increase blood flow to the brain, which allows the memory-making areas to work better.

> People who drank three or more glasses of fruit or vegetable juice a week cut their risk of dementia by over 75% compared with those who drank less than one weekly serving. Why not try dark grape juice? In a recent analysis of 59 fruits and veggies, black grapes were among those with the highest antioxidant capacity. Grapes may also help fight high blood pressure, cholesterol, diabetes, and cancer.

Blueberries also pack a powerful antioxidant punch. That's why researchers think this tiny fruit helps stave off diseases of aging, like Alzheimer's and Parkinson's. Antioxidants boost communication between neurons in your brain, improving movement-related skills and perking up your memory.

Cherries challenge high blood pressure. Gout sufferers have long turned to tart cherries for their anti-inflammatory properties. But did you know this tasty, popular fruit has also been found to improve memory?

A study of 34 generally healthy seniors found that those who drank 2 cups of Montmorency tart cherry juice a day for three months got better accuracy scores on memory and strategy tests than volunteers who drank a placebo.

"Cognitive function is a key determinant of independence and quality of life among older adults," says Sheau Ching Chai, assistant professor of behavioral health and nutrition at the University of Delaware and lead author of the study.

Chai says the improved scores may be related to the blood-pressure lowering effects of the anti-inflammatory compounds in tart cherries.

Studies suggest high blood pressure can lead to difficulties with memory, language, thinking, and judgment.

Hot drinks really warm up your memory

One sharp cookie. Doesn't miss a trick. Quick on the uptake. Do these phrases still describe you, or do you feel like your brain is veering off memory lane?

It's not too late to get back on track. Naturally occurring compounds in these beverages may help you remember things more easily.

Cocoa flavanols fire up thinking skills. Over age 60? If so, you might consider drinking hot chocolate every day. That may well be the advice of Italian researchers who studied the effects of cocoa flavanols on 90 healthy seniors.

Flavanols are compounds linked to your body's production of nitric oxide, a molecule that signals your blood vessels when they need to widen. That's important, say, during exercise when your muscles require increased supplies of oxygen- and nutrient-rich blood.

At the start of the study, the scientists tested the seniors' memory and reasoning skills. Then they randomly asked the volunteers to drink cocoa with either high, low, or medium amounts of flavanols each day.

- After eight weeks, the participants who drank the higher amounts of flavanols showed significant improvements in their memory and thinking. One possible reason? The extra flavanols — and additional nitric oxide — may have boosted blood flow to the brain.

- Interestingly, those volunteers also experienced improved blood pressure and reduced insulin resistance, a problem that leads to high blood sugar. Both are linked to brain health.

Time to give ginkgo the heave-ho

Thinking of buying *ginkgo biloba* supplements to improve your memory? You might want to reconsider. Mounting evidence suggests you'd be embarking on a fool's errand.

Studies show that gingko doesn't help prevent or slow dementia or cognitive decline, according to the National Center for Complementary and Integrative Health (NCCIH). Nor is there strong evidence that it improves memory in healthy people, says the NCCIH, a division of the National Institutes of Health.

Furthermore, ginkgo supplements can increase your risk of bleeding and cause headaches, stomach upset, and allergic skin reactions.

Still not convinced about over-the-counter ginkgo? The U.S. Government and Accountability Office reported in 2018 that it had tested two products marketed as ginkgo-containing, memory-boosting supplements. One had no gingko and the other had lower amounts than advertised.

Caffeine in coffee supports long-term recall. A Johns Hopkins University study suggests caffeine strengthens your brain's ability to convert short-term memories into long-term ones. Researchers recruited 160 adults who normally drank only small amounts of caffeine and asked them to study various pictures. The volunteers then either took a pill containing 200 milligrams of caffeine — about the same amount as in 2 cups of coffee — or a placebo.

The following day all the participants were tested on their ability to recognize images from the day before. Some of the photos were the same, others were new additions, and some were similar to the ones shown the previous day — say, a picnic basket with one handle instead of two.

There was no difference between the participants in their ability to identify previously seen and unseen pictures. But those who took the caffeine pill were significantly better at correctly identifying similar photos.

The researchers say the results may be caused by caffeine's ability to block reception of adenosine, a chemical that slows nerve center activity and makes you feel drowsy. The end result? Coffee makes you feel more alert and potentially improves your ability to process and store memories.

A long-term study of nearly 400 seniors found that those with low levels of vitamin D experienced cognitive decline up to three times faster than those who got enough of this important vitamin. But think twice before you up your D by adding cow's milk to coffee. Studies show mixing dairy proteins with phytonutrients may lower antioxidant activity.

2 power foods help you eat away forgetfulness

Best friends Shirley and Jenny shared a joyful reunion after a 23-year separation. Sweet, but not unheard of. So what makes their relationship so special? Jenny and Shirley are elephants. Guess it's true. Elephants really never do forget.

If your memory makes you feel a little "dumbo," try adding these two power foods to your menu. They're guaranteed to send you — and your super brain — right to the front of the herd.

To hook a better brain, think like Dr. Seuss. Remember reading the popular children's book *One Fish, Two Fish, Red Fish, Blue Fish* when you were a youngster? Bet you didn't know there's more to this title than meets the eye. Turns out both the redfish — aka the sockeye salmon — and the bluefish — a popular game fish found along the eastern seaboard — contain generous amounts of memory-boosting omega-3 fatty acids. These powerful nutrients defend your health in two delicious ways.

- Just one 3.5-ounce serving of fish — that's about the size of your checkbook — each week can keep your brain sharp and fight forgetfulness. Fatty fish like salmon, sardines, herring, and tuna are rich in the omega-3 fatty acids that protect your brain by getting rid of harmful beta-amyloid, a protein linked to Alzheimer's disease.

- Treat yourself to two delish fish feasts a week. This common food can help you live longer by fending off heart disease and high blood pressure — two conditions associated with memory loss. Omega-3 fatty acids to the rescue again. By keeping your blood from becoming sticky and forming clots, these little powerhouses can help stop a stroke in the making. Fish is also rich in calcium and vitamin D, two nutrients that fight weak bones.

Memory blurry? Try some curry. Dig into this delicious, spicy dish to protect your brain as you age. Turmeric, the bright yellow spice that gives curry powder its appealing color, contains curcumin. This compound helps stop one of the hallmarks of Alzheimer's disease — plaque buildup in the brain.

And researchers think curcumin improves your memory in more ways than one. "It may be due to its ability to reduce brain inflammation, which has been linked to both Alzheimer's disease and major depression," says Dr. Gary Small, director of geriatric psychiatry at the University of California, Los Angeles, and author of a recent study that shows curcumin supplementation boosts brainpower.

You can buy curcumin supplements, but the jar of turmeric spice you see at the grocery store may work just as well. Add 1/4 teaspoon of turmeric to your favorite recipes every day. And since your body doesn't absorb curcumin very well, help it out by pairing the turmeric with a little black pepper. Piperine, a substance found in black pepper, helps your body absorb more of the brain-booster.

Sardines: An unsung hero in a can

Feeling down in the dumps? Sardines are probably the last thing on your mind. But they shouldn't be. Sardines are loaded with healthy fats — omega-3 fatty acids — that have been linked to both improved mood and memory.

Aren't quite sure how to eat the silvery fish? Try these ideas for a nutritious, mind-boosting snack or meal.

- Pile on crunchy toast with a sliced tomato, red onion, or avocado.

- Broil or grill whole sardines. Squeeze lemon juice over the fish and garnish with fresh cilantro before serving.

- Mash into a paste before whisking into tomato sauce for extra flavor.

You can also add sardines to salads, use them in fish tacos, and toss them into pasta and rice dishes.

Score a touchdown at the table with these memory maximizers

The vast majority of Americans skimp on their vegetables, according to the Centers for Disease Control and Prevention. In fact, just 9% get their recommended 2 to 3 cups per day.

But that's no justification for pushing peas around your plate. Vegetables are important sources of fiber, minerals, and vitamins, and they're generally low in calories. What's more, this terrific trio not only makes for a tasty supper but also appears to slow — even prevent — memory loss in seniors.

Leafy greens sharpen recall. New research will have you loading up on spinach, kale, and collards in short order. Scientists divided

960 seniors into five groups based on the amount of leafy greens they ate each day and then tested their memory and thinking skills over five years.

It turns out that those who ate the most leafy greens — around 1.3 servings a day, or a little more than half a cup of cooked greens — had significantly less cognitive decline than those who ate the least.

In fact, the seniors who ate one to two servings a day had a mental edge that made it appear as if they were 11 years younger than those who avoided the veggies. The scientists say leafy greens are a rich source of vitamin K, lutein, and folate, which may help ward off memory loss.

Mushrooms fight off forgetfulness. According to a recent Singaporean study of 663 seniors, mushrooms look bright for brain health. Participants who ate over two portions of cooked mushrooms a week — 3/4 cup to a serving — more than halved their chances of having mild cognitive impairment (MCI) compared with those who ate less than one serving a week. MCI, a condition that can eventually lead to Alzheimer's disease, comes with symptoms like forgetfulness and loss of language and attention span.

Researchers believe the results may stem from the high amounts of an amino acid found in all kinds of mushrooms. Dubbed ergothioneine, the compound's antioxidant and anti-inflammatory properties may work to protect your brain from cell damage.

Other compounds in mushrooms, the scientists say, may prevent the formation of protein-rich plaques and tangles that set up in the brains of people with Alzheimer's disease.

Sweet potatoes perk up your memory. This versatile veggie — whether sliced, boiled, baked, roasted, grilled, or mashed — is one of the most nutritious you can eat.

And it may be key to helping prevent memory loss, according to a South Korean study on senior dietary habits. Researchers discovered that older adults with normal memory and verbal skills ate significantly more sweet potatoes than seniors with memory and thinking problems associated with MCI.

Though sweet potatoes in Asia are slightly different than the ones in American supermarkets, they have a lot in common. They're all rich in fiber, potassium, vitamins, and antioxidants like beta carotene.

The South Korean scientists say the vegetable's relatively low glycemic index (GI) — a measure of how quickly your blood sugar rises after eating a food containing carbohydrates — may help control insulin resistance, a condition linked to an increased risk of memory loss.

The glycemic index of your sweet potatoes will vary based on your cooking method. For a low GI, boiling is best.

MIND-ful eating cuts dementia risk

The MIND diet, short for Mediterranean-DASH Intervention for Neurodegenerative Delay, is the brainchild of Dr. Martha Clare Morris and colleagues at Chicago's Rush University Medical Center.

Their study shows that the MIND diet — a mashup of the brain-boosting Mediterranean and DASH diets — reduces the risk of Alzheimer's disease better than the other two plans. And you may see results even if you don't follow the MIND diet to the letter.

But who wouldn't want to? This food plan features tasty good-for-your-brain favorites like vegetables, nuts, berries, beans, whole grains, fish, poultry, olive oil — even a little wine. You'll still need to limit unhealthy choices like fried foods, butter, red meat, and cheese. Check with your doctor to see if the MIND diet can help you eat your way to a healthier brain.

Food for focus: Walnuts will supercharge your brain

Ever notice how much a walnut resembles the human brain? Crack open the rock-hard shell and you'll find the walnut kernel covered in wrinkles and folds — just like your cerebral cortex. It's even divided into left and right hemispheres. No wonder the ancient Greeks named the walnut "karyon," from the root word for "head."

Oddly enough, this unlikely pair has more in common than appearance. Walnuts contain important phytochemicals and healthy fats necessary for brain health. Recent research even suggests that eating walnuts may help prevent memory loss.

Natural compounds block deposits in the brain. A recent study suggests that walnuts may stave off the development of Alzheimer's disease (AD). Scientists divided mice that were bred to have AD into three groups.

- One set ate a walnut-free diet every day.

- The other two groups ate daily meal plans that contained either 6% or 9% walnuts. For humans, that would be about 1 to 1 1/2 ounces of walnuts — or 12 to 20 halves — a day.

When checked 10 and 15 months later, the brains of the mice who ate walnuts showed much less oxidative stress than the brains of the mice on a walnut-free eating plan. The researchers believe the antioxidants in walnuts prevented free radicals — rogue molecules — from harming brain cells.

That's important because oxidative damage is linked to the formation of beta-amyloid protein, a major component of amyloid plaques found in the brains of people with Alzheimer's.

Just a handful boosts concentration. Scientists at UCLA have discovered that eating walnuts may improve memory, concentration, and the speed at which you process information.

The researchers studied the data on a large group of adults age 20 and older who took part in several National Health and Nutrition Examination surveys. They found that participants who ate walnuts performed consistently better on cognitive tests compared with those who didn't eat the nuts. The results held true regardless of factors like age, gender, and ethnicity.

Lead scientist Lenore Arab says it took less than half an ounce of walnuts a day — about six halves — for the walnut eaters to benefit.

"It is exciting to see the strength of the evidence," says Arab. "It isn't every day that research results in such simple advice — eating a handful of walnuts daily as a snack, or as part of a meal, can help improve your cognitive health."

Scientists are pleased to see results from such a realistic amount of food, but how is it possible?

- The high amounts of antioxidants in walnuts may have contributed to the results, the researchers say.

- Walnuts also contain a significant amount of alpha linolenic acid (ALA), a plant-based omega-3 fatty acid with heart and brain benefits. According to a recent study from university docs, ALA may also help block the production of those dangerous beta-amyloid proteins.

Menopause

Soy-based cuisine could ease your estrogen woes

When you said you wanted a smoking hot body, you probably weren't thinking menopause would be the answer. But after you've stopped menstruating for a solid year, you've entered "the change of life" where hot flashes, night sweats, mood swings, and weight gain all hang on rather unpredictable hormonal shifts. As normal and natural as this transition is, it can also be uncomfortable and unsettling for some women.

The hormone estrogen regulates your menstrual cycle and impacts your bones, brain, skin, and more. But your estrogen levels begin to drop in the years leading up to menopause. Although study results are mixed, many experts say eating phytoestrogens, estrogen-like compounds found naturally in some plants, may calm some menopausal symptoms.

The secret to relief may be in the soybeans. Soy-based food has health-promoting phytoestrogens called isoflavones. And studies show that women eating an Asian diet with more soy tend to have fewer menopausal symptoms, such as hot flashes and bone loss, compared to those eating Western diets.

Some researchers believe the benefits from isoflavones may be tied to your ability to produce a beneficial compound called equol after eating isoflavone-packed foods like soy.

Only 25% to 50% of people can make equol, but the ones who do seem to respond better to dietary interventions like phytoestrogens.

Eat

Soybeans	Tofu
Soy milk	Apples
Celery	Garlic
Mangoes	Melons

Avoid

Symptom triggers such as alcohol, caffeine, hot drinks, and spicy food

Foods high in fat and sugar

Estrogen tank low? Fill up on phytoestrogens. Many foods rich in phytoestrogens are part of a healthy diet. These include foods like garlic, soybeans, celery, sweet potatoes, apples, and coffee.

Studies have found that eating 25 to 50 milligrams of isoflavones a day is safe and in tune with a traditional Japanese diet. That's the amount you'll find in one to two servings of tofu or 1 to 2 cups of soy milk.

The bottom line? If you are in menopause, getting phytoestrogens from plants could potentially relieve some of your symptoms.

News flash: Don't sweat symptoms with these supplements

Supplements are as popular as ever. Many on the market claim to remedy bothersome menopausal symptoms like hot flashes and night sweats. But are they safe and effective?

Researchers believe isoflavones may be an appealing solution for women who can't or won't use hormone replacement therapy (HRT), a treatment linked to many side effects. And if you can't get enough naturally through food, supplements may be a good add-on.

Experts still need to decide the best dose, though studies show 40 to 50 milligrams of soy isoflavones daily may help relieve symptoms. Smaller doses two times a day may be even better than taking them all at once. The North American Menopause Society suggests you opt for a trial-and-error approach to see what works for you.

A recent study published in the *American Journal of Clinical Nutrition* advises women with a risk of breast cancer not to take soy supplements.

Coffee runs hot and cold for these common symptoms

Thomas Jefferson called coffee the favorite drink of the civilized world. Dave Barry labeled it a medical necessity. But when it comes to menopause, that cup of joe comes with both pros and cons. That's why you'll have to pay attention to your specific symptoms to see if it's a smart choice for you.

Fatigue, fog, and frenzy — be gone. Tiredness, brain fog, and mood shifts often plague women in menopause. Fortunately, coffee has lots of good-for-you compounds. Some have estrogen-like effects that go to work protecting your brain. Others help you focus and may boost your memory.

When you drink coffee in moderation — up to 12 ounces a day — it can help you feel more alert and less sleepy, often within 15 minutes and for up to six hours.

Head off hot flashes. In a study of 1,806 women at the Mayo Clinic, one particular compound, caffeine, was linked to more hot flashes.

"While these findings are preliminary, our study suggests that limiting caffeine intake may be useful for those postmenopausal women who have bothersome hot flashes and night sweats," says Stephanie Faubion, M.D., director of the Women's Health Clinic at Mayo Clinic in Rochester.

To manage symptoms, she recommends you be aware of other triggers, such as spicy foods and hot beverages, and limit alcohol and tobacco.

Forego flatulent flare-ups. Gas and bloating can be embarrassing and unpleasant symptoms of menopause. Unfortunately, coffee, particularly the hot-brewed variety, is acidic. That can cause all sorts of problems like heartburn and upset stomach. Avoiding coffee or sticking to cold brews could save your stomach the irritation.

Shopping for milk: How to make the right 'moove'

Remember carefree days when you could guzzle a cup of milk, sport a mustache, and never once think of calories, fat, or sugar? You've still got good reasons to drink milk during menopause, but the type you choose should be based on your changing nutritional needs.

Whether it's from a cow, goat, nut, soybean, rice, or oat, your milk's nutrition label can help.

- Pay attention to "weighty" ingredients. For example, unsweetened plant-based milks often have fewer calories and less sugar than cow's milk. Control your portion by pouring the recommended serving size.

- Calcium supports bone health. So if you choose plant-based varieties, look for ones fortified with calcium carbonate. Studies show your body can absorb this kind as well as the calcium from cow's milk.

- Consider opting for soy-based milks, which are naturally packed with isoflavones, to control symptoms like hot flashes.

Grapes give menopausal women something to sing about

Have you heard through the grapevine that grapeseed extract — the product of the crushed seeds of red wine grapes — could ease your menopausal symptoms? It's true. Here's why.

In a randomized, double-blind, placebo-controlled trial, researchers identified 91 women between 40 and 60 years old who had at least one menopausal symptom. Over an eight-week period, the women took either 100 or 200 milligrams of grapeseed extract or a placebo.

Results showed that proanthocyanidins — the compounds that give grapes their color — did wonders.

- improved menopausal symptoms, including hot flashes and insomnia, in the high-dose group

- relieved anxiety, boosted muscle mass, and lowered blood pressure in the high- and low-dose groups

You can find grapeseed extract as a supplement in liquid or pill form in drugstores or online. It can cost between $7 and $47 a bottle.

Sweet treats beat midlife heat in a flash

Can't stand the heat? Get into the kitchen — and slice open a fresh, juicy pineapple. It's one of five fruits that may help cool off miserable hot flashes and night sweats.

Australian researchers discovered that women who ate the most fruit-rich diet had 20% less risk of hot flashes and night sweats than those who ate the least. This diet included apricots, strawberries, pineapples, melons, and mangoes.

If you can't really handle eating a lot of fruit right now, no problem. Another group of women cut their risk of hot flashes and night sweats by just as much as the fruit lovers, the researchers say. These women ate a Mediterranean-style diet with plenty of garlic, salad greens, peppers, mushrooms, pasta, and red wine.

Women who ate the most high-fat foods and sweets actually had more risk of hot flashes and night sweats. You may fit this high-fat-and-sugar profile if you eat a lot of cakes, meat pies, cookies, jam, and chocolate.

Osteoarthritis

Call on this veggie superfood to soothe your aching joints

Does every morning start with a snap, crackle, and pop? No, not from your breakfast cereal, but from your chatty joints. Those chronic noisy knees could be an early warning that you have a higher risk for osteoarthritis (OA), says a new study. But what exactly is OA?

Your skeleton has a natural cushion, called cartilage, that keeps your bones from rubbing and scraping together. Over time, this cartilage can wear away. And without that protection, your joints suffer from painful swelling and stiffness.

That's why this damage, better known as osteoarthritis, is often called a wear-and-tear disease. Age is a major risk factor, though old injuries and genetics also play a role.

Fortunately, you can help protect yourself with one food — broccoli. This common veggie can ease joint stiffness, cut pain, protect cartilage, and battle arthritis.

Surprising source of vitamin C wards off joint pain. You might be tempted to reach for an orange to boost your vitamin C. But leafy green veggies are a great way to get this nutrient, too. A single cup of raw broccoli clocks in with a whopping 81 milligrams (mg) — more than you'd get in a small orange.

Taiwanese researchers think this vitamin could be exactly what you need to head off OA. Past research shows that eating more vitamin C-rich

Eat

Broccoli	Turmeric
Ginger	Legumes
Cayenne pepper	
Green-lipped mussels	

Avoid

Soda
Pasta
White bread
White potatoes

foods can lower your risk of cartilage loss and arthritis. Experts think it's because this nutrient can help your body build more collagen, the tough connective tissue that helps protect your joints.

Exactly how much you need isn't quite clear to scientists yet, so for now it's best to stick with the daily recommended doses. Men should get around 90 mg, while women require 75 mg. If you want a break from broccoli, other foods like kale, spinach, bell peppers, and kiwis are outstanding sources, too.

Give your knees some broccoli love. Vitamin K is one of the most important nutrients for your skeleton and cartilage. Run low, and your bones and joints start to break down, causing the aches and pains of arthritis.

A recent study conducted by researchers at Tufts University revealed just how powerful this nutrient can be. Scientists studied 716 seniors over six to 10 years and found that people who had the least amount of vitamin K in their blood were also the likeliest to develop knee pain and mobility problems.

Fortunately, broccoli is chock-full of vitamin K. Add a cup of this chopped cruciferous veggie to your dinner plate for a boost of 92.5 micrograms. You'll be good for the day if you're a woman, but men will have to eat another third of a cup to meet their daily requirement.

Protect your cartilage with a helping of sulforaphane. Broccoli's arthritis-fighting powers aren't only due to vitamins. In fact, experts think this plant is loaded with unique ingredients that can save your cartilage from wearing away.

Sulforaphane, a naturally occurring compound, has been proven to block the enzymes that cause your joints to break down by stopping a key molecule that causes inflammation.

In a recent study, British researchers divided up 40 people with OA who needed knee replacements. Half were asked to eat a diet high in glucosinolates — the chemicals in broccoli that form sulforaphane — while the others were told to avoid them.

After two weeks, the scientists detected isothiocyanates (ITCs) — a breakdown product of glucosinolates — in the joints of those eating that diet, while the other group had none. The ITCs produced positive changes in the joint tissue, and scientists are hopeful future research will prove these compounds can help keep your cartilage healthy.

Save the stems to make the most of your broccoli

You wouldn't throw away a perfectly good apple, would you? But you probably don't think twice about tossing your broccoli stems in the trash after trimming off the florets. Not only is that a waste of money, you're missing out on vitamin C, fiber, iron, and other healthful nutrients.

With a little know-how, the broccoli stalk can be a nutritious, tasty treat that's every bit as good as the florets.

All you need to do is peel away the tough, outer layer. Underneath the woody skin, you'll find a light green, crisp layer that's great raw or cooked. Slice the stem into thin matchsticks, and they make the perfect addition to coleslaw, salads, or stir-fries.

Curb your arthritis pain with 3 powerful plants

Spices used to be worth their weight in gold. In fact, the Bible says when Queen Sheba visited King Solomon in 1,000 B.C. she offered him many spices in addition to gold and precious stones.

These days, the spices in your pantry aren't worth quite as much. But they're still valuable, especially if you have arthritis. These three common ingredients could be the key to warding off those crippling aches and pains.

Fight fire with flavor — spicy ginger could soothe your soreness.
When you're looking for relief and relaxation, fiery foods usually
don't top the list. But you might want to reconsider with ginger.
Scientists think it could be a great natural way to fight back
against your inflamed joints.

Researchers reviewed five studies that tested ginger's painkilling
power in a recent meta-analysis published in *Osteoarthritis and
Cartilage*. They found that taking 500 to 1,000 milligrams (mg) of
ginger extract daily blunts osteoarthritis pain and reduces disability
better than a placebo.

Experts think this remedy was so effective because ginger acts just
like over-the-counter NSAIDs such as aspirin and ibuprofen. It blocks
chemicals called leukotrienes and cyclooxygenase that cause inflammation and pain.

You can find ginger extracts online or at your local markets. If you
take blood thinners, talk to your doctor before starting supplements.

Turmeric tones down your pain. Are you sick of spending your
golden years dealing with the aches of arthritis? All you need is a
tiny pinch of turmeric to treat arthritis and inflammation.

Researchers conducted a systematic review of studies on turmeric
extract and its role in preventing OA pain. They found that taking
about a gram of curcumin — the powerful, naturally occurring
chemical in turmeric — every day for eight to 12 weeks offered the
same pain relief results as over-the-counter drugs. How? Curcumin
helps fend off oxidative stress and inflammation that causes swelling
and discomfort.

Even better? Experts say this spice can help protect your vision,
battle heart disease, and save your memory.

While turmeric doesn't have major side effects, it can still cause
stomachaches and digestive discomfort in large doses. You should
talk to your doctor before taking supplements or eating large amounts
of this spice.

Bring the heat of cayenne to cool your joints. Flaming hot jalapenos and blistering habaneros might not be a staple on your dinner table, but chances are you've got a bottle of cayenne pepper in your spice cabinet. And did you know that all three of these share the same active ingredient?

Capsaicin, the chemical that gives peppers their fiery burn, can do more than add pep to your plate. Experts say it can fight against sinus congestion, psoriasis, achy muscles, blood sugar spikes, belly fat, and poor blood circulation. And best of all? It can soothe your joints.

Not a fan of spicy food? Don't worry — you don't even have to eat cayenne to harness its pain-relieving powers. You simply need to rub it onto your skin.

A recent analysis of 17 studies revealed that topical capsaicin creams are just as effective at battling arthritis pain as over-the-counter drugs.

Before you go all in on these capsaicin-based treatments, rub a small amount on your skin to make sure it doesn't cause any irritation. Be extra careful to avoid getting it in your eyes and mouth, too.

Natural remedies give you a fighting chance

You can wash your hands 20 times a day, avoid crowded places, and still catch the flu. That's why you should get a flu shot every year — to give your body a little extra protection.

The same idea holds true for supplements. Even if you eat right, you may not get everything you need from food alone. These three supplements can give you added ammunition in your fight against arthritis.

Go "ananas" to attack inflammation and swelling. After Christopher Columbus brought the *Ananas comosus* — or pineapple as English-speakers called it — back to Europe, the tasty treat was so sought after that it could cost thousands of dollars. In fact, people would rent the fruit from vendors and return it uneaten, just so they could show off.

But as exotic as pineapples look, it's what's inside that makes them priceless. Bromelain, a naturally occurring enzyme in pineapple, may fight inflammation and swelling in your joints to ward off pain.

To see if this natural remedy could keep up with popular painkillers, scientists put it to the test. In a small study, 40 people with knee OA took either 500 milligrams (mg) of bromelain or 100 mg of the NSAID diclofenac. After four weeks, both treatments were equally effective at improving three measurements — pain, stiffness, and ability to perform daily activities like taking the stairs and getting out of a car.

Mythbuster: Do nightshades fire up symptoms?

Tomatoes always get the short end of the stick. In the 1700s, Europeans dubbed them "poison apples" because so many people got sick after eating them. In reality, the sickness was caused by the pewter plates aristocrats used.

Now, hundreds of years later, tomatoes and other nightshade vegetables still get a bad rap. Some people actively avoid them because they think these foods will worsen their arthritis symptoms. But how could veggies lead to throbbing knuckles and knees?

Nightshade plants contain solanine. Some people believe this chemical causes inflammation and arthritis pain. But research doesn't support this link. Experts say eating tomatoes, eggplants, bell peppers, and white potatoes shouldn't be a problem unless you have a food sensitivity.

Instead, most recommend adding more nightshades to your diet. These veggies are loaded with antioxidants and other nutrients that can help your fight against osteoarthritis.

Shore up your joints with a natural remedy. Feel a cold coming on? You might reach for a bowl of piping hot chicken soup. But do you know what to grab if your knees and knuckles are aching from arthritis?

Scientists say a supplement made from chondroitin sulfate (CS) might do the trick. This chemical is a building block of cartilage, so experts think adding it to your diet could help fight off OA.

> When it comes to soothing your creaky knees and aching hips, supplements pack a powerful punch. They provide nutrients and other natural compounds that can build up your joints and ease your suffering. Just remember they can interact with medications or cause complications if you have health problems. Always talk to your doctor before adding a new one to your medicine chest.

Recently, European researchers tested this theory. They enlisted 604 people with osteoarthritis in their knees, all 50 or older. Participants either took a placebo, a prescription NSAID, or an 800-milligram chondroitin sulfate supplement. After six months, they found that CS supplements were just as effective at fighting knee pain as the drugs. Both worked significantly better than the placebo.

Take advantage of a powerful "D"-fense against knee pain. Your body absorbs sunlight and turns it into vitamin D, which is an essential nutrient for a healthy skeleton. Scientists have found evidence that suggests high doses of this nutrient can support your joints, too.

Researchers in Thailand asked 175 people with osteoarthritis and low levels of vitamin D to take 1,000 micrograms (mcg) of vitamin D every week for six months. Not only did they raise their blood levels of this critical vitamin, they reported less joint pain, better muscle strength, and an improved quality of life.

Unfortunately, 1,000 mcg is a lot more than you can get through diet alone. You'd have to eat almost 5 1/2 pounds of herring just to come close. This is one time where a supplement will provide a bigger bang for your buck. Be sure and ask your doctor about the right amount for you.

The 'glue' you need to keep your joints healthy

People first tapped into collagen's powers thousands of years ago when ancient civilizations boiled animal bones to create glue. It was such a common practice that the protein responsible for the binding action was eventually named collagen, after the Greek word for glue.

An appropriate namesake, even in the medical world, because collagen gives your body structure and holds it together. It's even found in connective tissues like cartilage which helps support and cushion your joints. Now, scientists think collagen could change the way you fight off joint pain.

Stay independent with daily tasks. In a study published in *Nutrition Journal*, experts divided volunteers with osteoarthritis into one of three groups. They either got a collagen supplement, a placebo, or a dose of a common arthritis-fighting supplement called glucosamine hydrochloride plus chondroitin sulfate (GC).

After 180 days, scientists found that the people who took collagen had less knee pain and stiffness, compared to those who got the placebo or GC. The collagen group also reported greater improvements in their ability to perform daily tasks like putting on socks, shopping, and doing household chores.

Collagen tells aches to back off. So how does it work? You know damaged cartilage plays a huge role in osteoarthritis pain. But did you know that when your immune system responds to your damaged joints, it releases chemicals that can break down your cartilage even further?

That's where collagen comes in. Undenatured type II collagen (UC-II), the kind taken in this study, gradually teaches your immune system to leave your joints alone.

If you want to try this remedy at home, look for a 40-milligram daily supplement of UC-II. You can find it at health food stores or even online.

Flex these 'mussels' to fend off OA

Unless you've been living under the sea for the past 50 years, you've heard the buzz about fish oil. Among its many talents is the ability to help ward off arthritis pain, thanks to its omega-3 fatty acids.

But there's another source of joint-saving oil on the block — mussels, specifically green-lipped mussels native to New Zealand. Also known as the Greenshell mussel, this particular mollusk is loaded with two omega-3s — docosahexaenoic acid (DHA) and eicosapentaenoic acid (EPA) — that are proven inflammation fighters.

Recently, scientists put green-lipped mussels to the test in a small animal study. They found that adding a powdered version of this shellfish to the animal's diet could slow the progression of early, obesity-related osteoarthritis. The food was even more effective at blocking inflammation than over-the-counter medications.

If you can't find these mussels in your local supermarket, consider taking a supplement instead. You can buy green-lipped mussel supplements in most grocery stores or online.

The diet secrets that will save your knees

Have you ever put bad gas in your car? It will run, but you won't get the best performance out of your engine. Your diet is not that different. If you eat the wrong foods, you run the risk of creating problems. Fortunately, these easy steps are all it takes to avoid filling up your body with the wrong fuel.

Need to curb your pain? Cut out carbs. You know that sweet drinks can spike your blood sugar, but did you know a can of soda could cause your knees to ache? How about a plate of mashed potatoes?

Recently, researchers studied how eating a diet rich in high-carb foods like potatoes, sodas, and white bread can affect your joints. They asked one group of seniors with knee arthritis to stick with their normal diet, and instructed another group to eat a low-carb diet.

After three months, the people who ate fewer carbs had less pain in their knees than those who didn't change the way they ate.

Scientists think this diet is so effective because it helps lower oxidative stress in your body, which in turn helps prevent pain in your joints. Plus an animal study revealed that diets high in sugar cause joint inflammation.

The tiny sesame seed may be a huge help when it comes to arthritis pain. A study showed that adding about a quarter cup to your diet every day could help fight off inflammation and pain. It's easy to add these tasty nuggets to your menu. Sprinkle them into salads or stir-fries, or mix them into your morning oatmeal.

What does that mean for you? Instead of loading your plate with pasta and breadsticks, try eating more lean meats, fish, and vegetables.

Feast on fiber to dodge arthritis. You might worry about getting enough fiber if you skip bread, pasta, and rice. But don't worry — plants are loaded with it, too. Beans, legumes, and leafy greens are all outstanding sources of fiber. And that's great news for your joints.

A recent study of over 6,000 people found that those who ate the highest amount of fiber were much less likely to develop arthritis over a nine-year period than low-fiber eaters.

"Changing diets by increasing intake of dietary fiber seems to be one of the most economic ways to reduce the risk of knee osteoarthritis," says Dr. Zhaoli Dai, lead author of the study.

If your diet is a little low on roughage, start by adding a bowl of oatmeal to your breakfast menu and snacking on more fruits and veggies. Men should aim to get around 30 grams of fiber a day, while women need 21 grams.

And don't forget the beans and legumes. A single cup of tiny cooked lentils clocks in at 15.6 grams, half of what you need for the day.

Osteoporosis

'Bone' appétit: Turn to 2 Mediterranean staples for strength and support

They say your body is a temple. But if you don't want it ending up like the ruins in Greece, take a page out of a Greek recipe book instead. The Mediterranean diet, drawn from traditional Greek and Italian food, will give you nutrients to keep your bones strong.

Every day, cells called osteoclasts eat away at your bones. Normally, it's not a problem. Your body breaks down your bones to release minerals it needs — like calcium and phosphorus — into your bloodstream. Then it repairs the damage with a crew of rebuilding cells called osteoblasts.

Osteoblasts use the nutrients you eat to rebuild your skeleton as quickly as possible. Unfortunately, this process slows down as you get older, and you lose more bone than you make. If you don't get enough of the nutrients you need for rebuilding, like calcium and vitamin D, your bones become weak and brittle. This severe bone loss is called osteoporosis.

But don't let it diminish you. Luckily, the Mediterranean diet has your back and is putting minerals right into it. Add these two staples to your menu to give your bones a boost.

This snack is legen-dairy for its bone-strengthening traits. Yogurt is one of the most important foods you can keep in your fridge. That's because it's loaded with calcium. Your body uses this common mineral

Eat

Yogurt	Olive oil
Dried plums	Leafy greens
Chia seeds	Fish
Soy	Coffee
Tea	Turmeric

Avoid

Drinks with phosphoric acid, like soda

to fight high blood pressure, forgetfulness, and — you guessed it — weak bones.

In fact, calcium is one of the best nutrients you can enlist in your war against osteoporosis. About 99% of your body's calcium is stored in your bones where it supports and strengthens your frame. But your body will steal the mineral from your skeleton if you start running low.

Experts say you need to eat plenty of calcium to keep your bones strong, especially as you get older. You can get almost half of your daily needs in an 8-ounce container of low-fat yogurt.

You may be surprised to hear that having too much calcium or magnesium can hurt your manganese levels. Luckily, a deficiency is rare, but an extremely low intake may be damaging to your bones. Keep your manganese reserve up with foods like whole grains, legumes, tea, and spices.

Olive oil provides the support you need. Extra-virgin olive oil, which has the fun abbreviation EVOO, is a go-to in the kitchen. It tastes great and has the "bone"-us of being excellent for your skeleton.

One of EVOO's greatest powers against bone breakage is blocking the creation of those destructive osteoclasts. Certain polyphenols in the oil help minimize bone loss and keep your frame sturdy.

Even better, EVOO's polyphenols stimulate the bone-building osteoblasts to rapidly reproduce. They help preserve and repair your frame — no scaffolding required.

These protein powerhouses give calcium a boost

What's the most important nutrient you need to build your bones? If you guessed calcium, you get a gold star. But what you may not know is that calcium needs a team to keep your bones healthy and strong.

Protein is one of those key players. Scientists used to think too much protein was bad for your bones, but now studies suggest it is not harmful and may even have positive effects. One study examining calcium and protein intake found that vegans — people who don't eat meat or dairy — with low levels of calcium had a greater risk of fractures than meat eaters.

Researchers believe that eating more than the recommended 46 to 56 grams of protein daily — from both animal and vegetable sources — may help prevent bone loss as long as you also get enough calcium. Soy and fish are two protein-rich foods with nutrients that help you soak up calcium.

Dill-icious bone-strengthening sauce

The right foods can keep osteoporosis at bay, and Greek yogurt and olive oil make the perfect pair. Use them to make an easy dill sauce and stop your bones from crumbling away.

To get started, put 1 cup of Greek yogurt into a bowl. Stir in 1/4 cup of chopped dill, 1 teaspoon of lemon juice, and 2 teaspoons of olive oil. Grate 1 large garlic clove and add that before mixing them all together. Sprinkle in salt and black pepper to your liking and stir again. Finish with another pour of olive oil on top for a sleek finale.

Serve this sauce over your favorite fish, and you'll add a good dose of bone-building vitamin D.

Skipping out on soy could be a bone-breaking mistake.
Osteoporosis likes to play favorites. Unfortunately, women are more likely to wind up with brittle bones than men. There are a few reasons — women live longer so the disease has more time to set in, plus their bones tend to be smaller and lighter. But most of the blame lies with a hormone called estrogen.

Once menopause sets in, your body doesn't make as much estrogen — which is a big problem. This hormone plays a huge part in slowing bone breakdown and helping your body hang on to calcium.

That's where soy comes in. It's loaded with natural chemicals called isoflavones that look a lot like estrogen. They are so similar your body has trouble telling them apart, which means they can help your bones absorb calcium, just like naturally occurring estrogen does.

* In a small study published in the *American Journal of Clinical Nutrition*, researchers pitted soy isoflavones against one of the top-rated osteoporosis drugs on the market.

* While the soy supplements didn't quite match the results of the drugs, the most effective dose — 105 milligrams (mg) of soy isoflavones — was still considered a success in helping bones hold on to calcium. And it worked without the dangerous side effects that come with medications.

Experts say 50 to 100 mg of soy isoflavones every day may be enough to improve your bone health. You can get 56 mg in a half cup of boiled soybeans. Mix up your menu with other high-isoflavone foods like edamame, tofu, tempeh, and miso.

Reel in this superfood to double down on your skeleton. Fish swim in schools because they understand the value of sticking together. And just like them, the nutrients in your body can't work alone. One of calcium's biggest supporters is vitamin D.

Your body can make vitamin D all by itself, just by soaking up sunlight. But as you get older, this process slows down, so you need to get more of the nutrient from your diet. Fortunately, there's a tasty treat loaded with the stuff — salmon. One can of sockeye salmon with the bones delivers well over 100% of your daily recommended dose.

But that's not all this fatty fish has to offer. That same salmon is packed with omega-3 fatty acids — another osteoporosis fighter for your arsenal. Here's the lowdown.

- In a recent study, experts looked at the diets of 1,865 women in Spain. They found that those who ate the most omega-3 also had the strongest bones in their hips and lower backs.

- The scientists think omega-3 curbs chronic inflammation that contributes to the development of osteoporosis.

The 'it' fruit and vegetable to fight osteoporosis

If you have trouble keeping track of all the bone-boosting foods out there, just remember these two — spinach and dried plums, aka prunes. With the help of vitamin K, they make skeletal strengthening simple.

Leaf those brittle bones behind. Studies show that a shortage of vitamin K1, which is found in leafy greens like spinach and cabbage, is linked to a higher risk for fractures.

Experts noticed something interesting, though. When people with brittle bones bulked up on this vitamin, they were a lot less likely to suffer a broken bone even though their bone density didn't improve. Researchers think it might have something to do with the way this nutrient improves the overall quality of your skeleton.

It's pretty easy to get, too. A cup of cooked spinach is packed with more than seven times your daily recommended dose. As an added bonus, you'll also get a quarter of your calcium needs.

Dried plums are the next superfruit, and they're great for your bones. Blueberries have rave reviews for their health benefits, but there's a new superfruit in town. It's cheap, sweet, and may already be in your fridge. Dried plums rival blueberries with how much disease-fighting power they have.

Like blueberries, dried plums are packed with antioxidants. But with the prunes, you can reach your fruit goals on a lower budget. If you eat a typical American diet, 2 cups of fruit are recommended per day.

But more may be better, according to a study published by the *American Journal of Clinical Nutrition*. Researchers reported that women who doubled their fruit intake increased their spine mineralization by 5%.

Dried plums in particular can outperform the competition. Just one serving, about five to six prunes, is enough to benefit your bones. In a study comparing one serving to two servings, researchers found that the smaller amount was just as effective in preventing bone loss in older postmenopausal women.

Women who eat five to six dried plums each day will get about a third of their daily recommended intake of vitamin K. Plus they'll benefit from the many polyphenols found in the fruit. Studies show those compounds help improve bone mass, too.

Best late-night snack for your bones

Don't ditch dessert in your pursuit of health. Chia seed pudding is the late-night goodie you can have guilt-free.

A small study of postmenopausal women with weakening bones, called osteopenia, found that a nighttime calcium supplement improved their bone formation and reduced bone loss. That's why chia pudding makes the perfect case for an evening treat. Chia seeds contain calcium, manganese, magnesium, and more.

Begin by whisking together 1/2 cup of milk, 1/2 cup of plain, low-fat Greek yogurt — to give you even more calcium — and 1/8 teaspoon of salt. Pick a sweetener, like honey or maple syrup, and stir in 1 tablespoon. Then add 1/4 cup of chia seeds, and mix all the ingredients together.

Leave your pudding to cool and thicken in the refrigerator overnight. When it's ready to eat, top with a few dried plums for extra flavor and a healthy chunk of vitamin K.

Hottest drinks for a healthy frame

What's better than a cup of coffee or tea to pep you up in the morning? The fact that a steamy sip of either can help secure your bone health.

Coffee beans are bone boosters. Orange juice may be the first thing that comes to mind when you think of acidic drinks, but coffee has acids in it, too. And lucky for you, they're good for your bones.

Caffeic acid, chlorogenic acid, and vanillic acid are just three of the acids found in your favorite cup of joe. Many of these acids behave like estrogen in your body. That means they can help improve bone mineral density and fight osteoporosis caused by an estrogen deficiency.

If a drink could melt your bones, it would be soda. More than two servings a day may increase the risk of hip fracture in postmenopausal women. That's because the caffeine and phosphoric acid in soft drinks can prevent your body from absorbing calcium. Watch out for colas in particular — they're the worst in the bunch.

The sweet spot is drinking 2 to 3 cups. In a recent study of postmenopausal women, those who drank 2 or 3 cups of coffee a day had a lower risk of fractures compared to women who drank less than 1 cup. But drinking 4 or more cups increased fracture risk.

Of course, drinking too much coffee has other drawbacks as well, like increased anxiety, headaches, and insomnia. So keep your intake in the moderate range to reap the most benefit.

Brew up a cup of tea to crack down on fractures. Feeling down in the dumps? A piping hot cup of tea is the perfect pick-me-up, but this old remedy can do more than help you feel better on a blustery day. Your tea leaves actually offer some serious protection for brittle bones.

In a recent meta-analysis, scientists pored over 13 studies that revealed just how powerful tea can be. The studies revealed people who drink tea tend to have stronger bones in their necks, lower backs, and hips than their non-tea-drinking counterparts.

The secret lies with a naturally occurring plant chemical in tea called epigallocatechin gallate (EGCG). It works by increasing the activity of osteoblasts, which are the cells your body uses to repair broken-down bones. And it helps the osteoblasts already in your body live longer and work harder.

The studies don't recommend a single type of brew, but green teas tend have the highest levels of EGCG, followed by white, oolong, and black teas. If better bone health is your cup of tea, start sipping today.

Probiotic power can save your skeleton

Your gut bacteria do everything from improving digestion to fighting off ailments. And a brand-new study shows that they can protect your frame, too.

German researchers split 70 older women with low bone mineral density into two groups. Half took a placebo, while the others got a powder packed with a probiotic supplement of *Lactobacillus reuteri*.

Among the women who took probiotics for a year, bone loss was slashed in half compared to women who received placebos. Experts think these friendly bacteria help your body keep inflammation in check. Plus they may block the overproduction of bone-eating cells.

People in the study took 10 billion colony-forming units (CFUs) of *L. reuteri* a day. If you want to try the same at home, track down probiotic supplements or yogurts with the same strain. If they aren't at your local grocery store, you can always head online.

Beware of anti-nutrients working against you

Some food bad guys are obvious. They're cloaked in a sugar coating or have an ingredient label that sets off as many alarm bells as a villainous monologue.

But what about when your vegetables, the heroes in your health story, turn against you? Anti-nutrients are compounds that can block the absorption of nutrients, and they're found in your favorite greens and legumes.

Several of these anti-nutrients impact your bones because they hurt calcium absorption. Oxalates in leafy greens and tea, and phytates in whole grains are two examples. But you don't want to give up on these foods because they offer so many other benefits. Here are some things you can do to lessen these compounds' effects.

- Stagger the times you eat foods with anti-nutrients. For example, try drinking tea between meals instead of with them. That way you can still absorb your meal's calcium.

- Boil or soak your food to remove anti-nutrients like lectins in legumes or glucosinolates in broccoli.

- Avoid eating large amounts of anti-nutients at the same meal. Instead, vary your diet throughout the day.

This spice will curry favor with your bones

By the time turmeric made it to America, people thought it was little more than a way to add some color and flavor to exotic curries. But scientists have begun to delve into the healing powers of this golden spice. Now new research has discovered that the active ingredient in turmeric — a naturally occurring chemical called curcumin — could hold the key to beating brittle bones.

In a recent Italian study, researchers split 57 people with low bone density into two groups. Half were told to exercise a few times a week and eat a diet with plenty of calcium, vitamin D, and vitamin C. The others got the same instructions plus a daily curcumin supplement of 1,000 milligrams.

At the end of the six-month study, people who took the supplement saw improvements in the bone density measurements of their fingers, heels, and upper jaws. The control group, on the other hand, didn't see significant changes. Scientists think it's because curcumin can actually slow down your body's production of bone-breaking osteoclasts.

The turmeric powder you'll find at the grocery store is about 3% curcumin, so to get the same amount measured in the study you'd need to wolf down about 11 teaspoons of the stuff daily. Eating that much turmeric every day could cause stomachaches or other digestive discomfort.

But you can track down supplements at your local market or online. Curcumin doesn't mix well with some medications like blood thinners, so talk to your doctor before taking supplements.

Prostate cancer

Triple threat — wash away your cancer risk with 3 powerful drinks

Did you know a man's risk of developing prostate cancer rises with age? Nearly 175,000 Americans are diagnosed with this devastating disease annually. Some 6 in 10 are seniors over age 65.

You may recall the prostate is a walnut-sized gland below a man's bladder. It surrounds part of the urethra, a tube that allows urine to pass from your body. Symptoms of prostate cancer include painful or frequent urination, lower backache, and discomfort during ejaculation.

Of course, there's no surefire way to avoid developing the disease. But science suggests these three drinks may cut your risk.

Call on coffee to keep cancer at bay. A recent study in the *International Journal of Cancer* found that men who drank 3 cups of Italian-style coffee daily — think espresso, cappuccino, or macchiato — were 53% less likely to develop prostate cancer than those who drank less than that. The exact reasons behind coffee's cancer-fighting powers aren't totally clear, but the researchers believe caffeine may play a role.

In a separate study, Japanese scientists discovered that two chemical compounds in coffee — kahweol acetate and cafestol — can slow the growth of transplanted prostate cancer cells in mice. Further testing is necessary to see if these findings can be applied to humans, but early research is promising.

Eat	
Coffee	Green tea
Rooibos tea	Mushrooms
Broccoli	Herring
Turmeric	Oregano
Red grape juice	Tofu
Whole-grain rye	

Avoid

Red meat like beef, pork, and lamb

Warning: High-dose vitamins could put you in danger

Supplements and vitamins that boast about beating back prostate cancer sound tempting. But these pills aren't always all they're cracked up to be.

In fact, recent research suggests some supplements might do more harm than good. Italian scientists discovered that high levels of vitamin E can cause cellular damage and may increase your risk of developing prostate cancer.

Instead of reaching for a bottle of vitamins, experts say you should get most of your nutrients from foods. Consult your doctor if you need extra help with your diet. He may be able to help you find a solution that doesn't increase your risk of cancer.

Go ape over grape's antioxidant powers. Research suggests that each glass of red wine you drink per week may lower your risk of prostate cancer by 6%. The same study showed that men who drank eight glasses of red wine a week reduced their risk of aggressive prostate cancer by 61%. One possible reason? Red wine is loaded with the antioxidant resveratrol, which may cause prostate cancer cells to self-destruct.

Of course, drinking too much alcohol can lead to a host of health problems, including heart and liver disease, pancreatitis, stroke, and several types of cancer. Fortunately, wine isn't your only source of resveratrol. Dark red and purple grape juice have the same powerful antioxidants.

Tap into tea for a catechin boost. Chinese researchers published an analysis in *Medicine* that links the drinking of more than 7 cups of green tea a day to a lower risk of prostate cancer. They say green tea is loaded with antioxidant compounds called catechins, which may keep prostate cancer from growing and spreading.

Not a big fan of green tea? Don't worry — you have another option. A recent animal study suggests an herbal tea, known as rooibos, can stop cancer cells from reproducing. The tests haven't been done on people yet, but keep your ear to the ground for more information.

You'll find rooibos tea at most supermarkets or you can order it online.

Try this superfood supper to slash your risk of cancer

Next time you order Chinese takeout, you might want to try a stir-fry with broccoli, tofu, and mushrooms. It's a savory supper packed with nutrients that may help you head off prostate cancer.

Mushrooms are must-haves for staying in tiptop shape. Japanese scientists tracked the diets and health of nearly 36,500 men for 13 years. After sifting through the data, they found a surprising superfood — mushrooms — that gives you an edge on this disease.

In fact, this humble vegetable is so packed with nutrients, just two servings a week is enough to reduce your risk of prostate cancer. Compared with men who ate mushrooms less than once a week, those who consumed the veggie once or twice a week lowered their risk by 8%. Eating mushrooms more often appeared to bring even bigger benefits. Those who ate at least three servings per week slashed their odds by 17%.

So what makes these little fungi so fantastic? Experts think the credit lies with an antioxidant in mushrooms called l-ergothioneine. This naturally occurring compound fights off oxidative stress, which can lead to cell damage and cancer. L-ergothioneine is found in shiitake and oyster mushrooms, but researchers say common white button mushrooms may have anti-cancer compounds, too.

Sup on soy to protect yourself. Researchers from the University of Illinois at Urbana-Champaign recently analyzed multiple studies on soy and discovered that men who ate a diet rich in unfermented soy products — like tofu and soy milk — were 30% less likely to get prostate cancer.

The reason lies with soy's isoflavones, chemical compounds that have estrogen-like effects. Sometimes called the female hormone, estrogen helps the prostate function normally. Researchers believe isoflavones bind to estrogen receptors in the prostate, which helps prevent cancer cells from forming and multiplying.

Cook up crispy tofu with this simple guide

With a little know-how, you can turn tofu into a tasty treat guaranteed to win over any meat-lover.

Start with a block of firm tofu. It absorbs flavors well and holds its shape during cooking better than the soft and silken varieties. Slice the tofu into bite-sized pieces and put them in a colander. Pour salted, boiling water over the tofu to draw out excess moisture. Let cool before blotting dry with a paper towel.

Place the pieces in a little bit of oil and your favorite spices before coating them in cornstarch. Arrange them in a single layer on a baking sheet, and roast in a 375-degree oven for 25 minutes, or until golden brown.

Voila! You're ready to dish up crispy tofu nuggets on their own, in a stir-fry, or with your favorite dipping sauce.

Beat back disease with help from broccoli. A compound in broccoli called sulforaphane may stop the spread of prostate cancer, according to a new study published in the *American Journal of Clinical Nutrition*.

Researchers recruited men who had slow-growing prostate cancer and asked them to eat a little over 1 1/4 cups of broccoli soup a week for a year. Some ate soup made from ordinary, run-of-the-mill broccoli. The rest had broccoli soup that contained either three or seven times the level of sulforaphane as the control soup.

Twelve months later, tests on the men who ate the soup with added sulforaphane showed suppression of a gene that causes cancer cells to spread. Those given the largest amount of the compound saw the best results.

The researchers say the men in the control group didn't get enough sulforaphane to see similar benefits. Fortunately, you can increase the amount you get by adding other cruciferous vegetables like Brussels sprouts, cabbage, and cauliflower to your diet.

Protect your prostate with this no-fuss nosh

Simplicity — a way of life in Scandinavia — is probably best represented by Denmark's classic, open-faced sandwich. Dubbed smørrebrød, it's a slice of lightly buttered rye bread often topped with pickled herring or smoked salmon. And believe it or not, this easy meal is packed with powerful protection for your prostate.

Swap the wheat for rye to stop the spread of cancer. In a small study, Swedish researchers asked men with prostate cancer to eat either whole-grain and bran rye products every day, or foods made from refined wheat with added fiber. After six weeks, the rye eaters showed signs of slower cancer growth in their prostates.

Experts credit rye's potent powers to plant compounds called lignans. Previous studies discovered that these nutrients increase your body's levels of endostatin — a naturally occurring protein that blocks cancer cells from growing and spreading.

Want to add lignans to your diet? The men in the study ate a little over a pound of food containing whole-grain or bran rye each day. That's about 15 slices of bread. Fortunately, you can also find rye in different types of cereal, porridge, and crackers. Flaxseeds, cashews, peanuts, broccoli, and apricots are rich sources of lignans, too.

Cut back on calcium to stay hale and hearty

Takeru Kobayashi is no stranger to extreme eating. He might be best known for downing 50 hot dogs in 12 minutes, but he also made headlines for chugging a gallon of milk in under 20 seconds.

Much as you might like milk, think twice before trying to break that record. Researchers claim men who get too much calcium in their diet are more likely to develop prostate cancer. They think it's because high levels of calcium can impact your body's ability to produce vitamin D.

Of course, that doesn't mean you should stop drinking milk entirely. Your body still needs some calcium to keep your bones healthy. And some studies suggest it may protect you against diabetes and high blood pressure.

Instead, try to keep your daily intake of calcium to around 1,200 milligrams. That's about what you'd get from 4 cups of milk.

Reel in this vital vitamin to amp up protection. Scientists from Arizona studied the diets of more than 1,650 men with prostate cancer. They discovered that those who got high amounts of vitamin D were less likely to have the high-risk form of the disease that requires more aggressive treatment.

The men in the study who most benefited got at least 15 micrograms (mcg) of vitamin D each day. You'd have to drink around 6 cups of milk to get that amount. Of you could eat herring. A single ounce of this fatty fish has a whopping 11.25 mcg.

Looking for other sources of this important nutrient? Try drinking more vitamin D-fortified orange juice and cereals.

Fill up on fish to get the right fats. A new study published in *Nutrients* examined the eating habits of men with slow-growing prostate cancer. Researchers found that those whose diets contained a lot of long-chain omega-3 fatty acids were less likely to develop the high-risk form of the disease. The researchers say omega-3s fight off inflammation in your prostate, which helps keep cancer from spreading.

Gentlemen, listen up. Do you normally order a burger or steak when you go out to eat? Experts say men are more likely to eat meat than women, a practice that could jeopardize your health. The World Health Organization says eating too much red meat may increase your risk of prostate cancer.

Be sure to get your fill of fatty acids by eating fish like herring, salmon, tuna, and sardines at least once a week.

Double down on flavor to turn up your defenses

Herbs and spices can do more than zest up your dinner. The right ones can give you an extra dose of cancer-fighting nutrients.

Sprinkle on this powerful herb for a heaping helping of protection. A single tablespoon of dried oregano packs more antioxidants than an entire apple. And experts think one antioxidant in particular — carvacrol — could help you fend off prostate cancer.

Studies suggest this powerful nutrient may stop prostate cancer cells from growing, and may even cause them to self-destruct. Carvacrol still needs to be tested on humans. But that doesn't mean you have to wait. A few dashes of oregano are all you need to spice up an otherwise bland meal.

Slow down cancer with this exotic spice. You may want to pick up some turmeric, the golden root that gives curry its vibrant color, next time you're in the produce aisle. That's because curcumin — the main antioxidant in this spice — may prevent the growth of prostate cancer.

Korean researchers recently put turmeric to the test.

- They asked men with prostate cancer to take a curcumin supplement or a placebo daily after they completed the first phase of their cancer treatment.

- At the end of six months, those who took curcumin had fewer signs of prostate-specific antigen (PSA) progression than the placebo group. Experts say that could be a sign their cancer growth had slowed.

Men in this study took 1,440 milligrams of curcumin every day. To get that through your diet alone, you'd need about 5 tablespoons of turmeric a day. That's a lot, so consider asking your doctor about taking a supplement. In the meantime, you can sprinkle this Indian spice onto veggies or into soups and smoothies.

Prostate problems

These nutritional superstars help you go with the flow

Do you wake up every few hours to take a trip to the bathroom? You're not alone. More than one-third of men have symptoms of an enlarged prostate by age 60, including frequent urination, streams that start and stop, and trouble emptying the bladder.

This condition — known as benign prostatic hyperplasia (BPH) — is a common part of getting older. But a poor diet can make your symptoms worse. Fortunately, these three foods may keep those nightly bathroom visits at bay.

Let garlic guard your prostate. Research suggests that a diet rich in garlic and onions decreases your risk of developing an enlarged prostate.

Why do these versatile veggies pack a powerful punch? Korean researchers offered up a theory after a four-week study of rats with BPH. The scientists fed the rats either garlic powder or medicine used to treat the disorder. Surprisingly, the garlic was just as effective at shrinking the prostate as the drugs.

The authors suggest garlic blocks inflammation-causing enzymes that can cause your prostate to become enlarged. They also believe garlic triggers the production of molecules that ensure damaged cells die in a timely manner. Further studies are needed to see if similar results occur in humans.

Eat	
Garlic	Tomatoes
Leafy greens	Sardines
Pumpkin seeds	Berries

Avoid
Coffee
Spicy foods
Alcohol

Tape your tomatoes to stop the rot

You've probably heard that you shouldn't store tomatoes in the refrigerator. That's because the cold temperature halts the enzyme activity responsible for flavor, texture, and color.

The only problem? Keeping ripe tomatoes on the kitchen counter means they'll likely go bad sooner. Fortunately, there's an easy solution. You can extend a tomato's shelf-life with a common household item — tape.

Find the spot on your tomato where the stem was cut from the vine. Cover it with tape to prevent water from leaving the tomato and to stop bacteria from finding their way in.

If a tomato isn't quite ripe when you bring it home, don't tape it right away. Store an unripe tomato upside down in a paper bag on your counter until it's nice and red.

Tuck into tomatoes to crush your risk. Who doesn't love the summer? This season brings sunny days, warm weather, and — best of all — ripe and juicy tomatoes fresh from the garden.

But tomatoes are more than a tasty addition to your salads. It turns out that the chemical compound that gives tomatoes their red color — a nutrient called lycopene — could help lower your risk of BPH.

Italian scientists sorted men with enlarged prostates into two groups. All of them had lower urinary tract symptoms caused by their condition. One group took a daily placebo, while the other took a supplement containing lycopene and other nutrients each day. After three months, the men who took the supplement showed signs that their prostate growth had slowed.

Get your greens to fight off infections. Chinese researchers who tracked the eating habits of elderly men for four years discovered that a diet rich in fruit and vegetables was linked to a lower risk of BPH. Dark and leafy greens offered up the most protection. Experts say these veggies are packed with nutrients — like vitamin C and beta carotene — that combat inflammation and oxidative damage.

The men in the study who saw the most benefits ate sufficient amounts of fruits and vegetables, including around 100 grams of dark and leafy veggies a day. You can get more than half of that in 2 cups of raw spinach.

Pass the sardines, protect the prostate

Sardines may be known as a cheap meal, but that wasn't always the case. In the past, these tiny fish were prized delicacies. The son of Irish playwright Oscar Wilde even launched a sardine-tasting club for high-society Londoners in the 1930s.

The idea of eating sardines may have lost its luster over the years, but you should still add them to your plate. They're packed with two nutrients that help keep your prostate in tiptop shape.

Pick the right fat to shrink your prostate. It's probably no surprise that a diet full of fatty foods like burgers and fries is linked to an increased risk of prostate problems. Fortunately, including the omega-3 fatty acids in fish can help ward off those woes.

Researchers prescribed identical drugs to 100 men who had lower urinary tract symptoms caused by BPH. Then they asked half of the men to take an omega-3 supplement along with their medication. Six months later, the men who took the supplement and the drug experienced more shrinkage in the size of their prostates than those who took only the medication.

The men in the study got 900 milligrams of omega-3 a day. You can get nearly that amount by eating five sardines.

Take a deep dive to get more of this delightful vitamin. Believe it or not, vitamin D technically isn't a vitamin. It's a hormone that's mostly produced in your skin when it's exposed to sunlight. But as you age, your body often doesn't make enough vitamin D to keep up with your needs. And that could put you at risk for prostate problems.

In a recent study, Chinese researchers examined the vitamin D levels in 322 elderly men and found that those who didn't have enough of this nutrient were more likely to have an enlarged prostate. Experts say vitamin D binds to the receptors in prostate cells, which helps protect you from inflammation and other causes of prostate cell growth.

Men over age 50 should get at least 15 micrograms (mcg) of vitamin D in their diet each day. That number jumps to 20 mcg if you're over age 70. Fatty fish are one of the best sources of this nutrient. A 3.75-ounce can of sardines, for example, provides you with 6.25 mcg.

> Need another excuse to crack open a can of sardines? These flavorful fish are packed with protein. A small tin of sardines provides nearly half of the protein you need each day. Researchers say eating more of this nutrient may lower your risk of an enlarged prostate.

Pile on the pumpkin seeds for a clean bill of health

Next time Halloween rolls around and you're carving a jack-o-lantern, think twice before throwing away the gooey insides of your pumpkin. Aside from being a tasty treat, those seeds are loaded with nutrients and minerals that could hold the key to fending off BPH.

Snack on seeds to snuff out inflammation. German researchers asked 1,431 men with BPH to take either a placebo, a capsule containing 500 milligrams (mg) of pumpkin seed extract, or a handful of pumpkin seeds twice a day for a year.

Twelve months later, the scientists discovered that the men who ate the pumpkin seeds had significant improvement in their symptoms compared with those who took the placebo or the extract. The scientists believe these results were caused by compounds in pumpkin seeds called sterols. These naturally occurring chemicals may help combat the chronic inflammation that can cause your prostate to become enlarged.

Want to try it yourself? Men in this study ate 10 grams of pumpkin seeds a day, which works out to about 2 1/2 tablespoons.

Skip the supplements — herbal products don't offer proven protection

Herbal supplements promise a lot when they claim the ability to shrink an enlarged prostate. Unfortunately, they don't keep up their end of the bargain.

Saw palmetto was once seen as a cure-all for prostate problems. But a study published in the *Journal of the American Medical Association* claims this herb is no more effective than a placebo.

Experts say one problem is that herbal supplements aren't closely regulated, so the ingredients listed on the label aren't necessarily in your pills.

The bottom line? Get your nutrients from food instead of wasting your hard-earned dollars on empty promises.

Don't miss out on this mighty mineral. You need zinc for lots of things — a strong immune system, cell division, and the ability to break down carbohydrates, for starters. And you may be at risk for BPH if you don't get enough of this trace mineral.

But be careful. Getting too much zinc through supplements has been linked to an increased risk of advanced prostate cancer. You should get 11 mg of this nutrient each day through zinc-rich foods like legumes, dark chocolate, and whole grains.

Nuts and seeds are other good sources. A half cup of pumpkin seeds, for example, will provide you with nearly 20% of that amount.

Overcoming impotence: 2 trusty solutions you need to try

Erectile dysfunction (ED) can be brought on by treatments for prostate cancer or medications for an enlarged prostate. It can also be caused by heart disease, high cholesterol, and obesity.

The good news? Dodging this dreaded condition can be as easy as changing what's on your dinner plate.

Fill up on fruit to boost your blood flow. Need another reason to add more fruit to your diet? A recent study published in the *American Journal of Clinical Nutrition* could convince you to snack on more apples, oranges, and berries.

Scientists analyzed the diets of more than 25,000 men and found that those who ate the most fruit had a 14% lower chance of having erectile dysfunction compared with men who ate the least amount of fruit. The reason lies with fruit's flavonoids. These naturally occurring compounds help relax your blood vessels, which makes it easier for you to get and maintain an erection.

Take a trip to the Mediterranean to battle back against ED. European researchers recently reviewed four studies that examined the link between the Mediterranean diet and erectile dysfunction.

This traditional eating plan, which emphasizes whole grains, nuts, vegetables, and healthy fats like olive oil, is a natural way to fend off bedroom woes. One possible reason? The antioxidant-rich Mediterranean diet provides your body with an amino acid called arginine. This compound raises nitric oxide production, which improves the blood flow needed for an erection.

Ditch the decaf to dodge erectile dysfunction

Cutting back on your morning cup of coffee may be a good idea if you have BPH. Caffeine, after all, increases your need to urinate. And that's bad news if your enlarged prostate is blocking the flow of urine from your bladder.

But you might think twice before switching to decaf. Researchers studied the coffee-drinking habits of more than 21,400 men. They found that those who had 4 or more cups of decaffeinated coffee per day had a 37% greater risk of erectile dysfunction than those who didn't drink it.

Experts aren't quite sure why that's the case. They say that micronutients and antioxidants might somehow get removed during decaffeination. Another possibility? Harmful chemicals might be added during the process.

Diet do's and don'ts to fend off infections

An enlarged prostate isn't the only reason for frequent, painful trips to the bathroom. Your symptoms could be caused by prostatitis. This condition — which causes your prostate to become inflamed and swollen — can be brought on by bacterial infections contracted, say, during a prostate biopsy or when using a urinary catheter.

Normally, these symptoms clear up after a few days or weeks. But sometimes the disease lingers for months. Fortunately, you might be able to find relief with a little help from your diet.

Pick probiotics to battle long-lasting bacteria. Want to keep prostatitis at bay? Give your immune system a helping hand. That's the advice of Italian researchers who found that probiotics — live yeast and bacteria that are good for you — can lower the risk of recurring prostatitis as well as help prevent the inflammation from spreading to other glands.

The scientists gave men with prostatitis and irritable bowel syndrome a round of antibiotics. Once their infections were under control, the men continued for one year to receive weekly medications along with a daily probiotic supplement or placebo. At the end of the study, the men who took the probiotic were significantly less likely to have infections in their prostates.

If you want to try this at home, the men took a probiotic called *VSL#3*, which is made up of eight strains of bacteria from the *Lactobacillus* and *Bifidobacteria* families. Talk to your doctor about taking a similar supplement. You can also get probiotics from yogurts and other naturally fermented foods and drinks.

Steer clear of trigger foods to soothe your symptoms.
Sometimes, the foods you avoid are just as important to your health as the ones you eat.

Researchers published a study in *Urology* that examined the diets of nearly 100 men with chronic prostatitis. They found that foods like hot peppers, coffee, chili, and alcohol made their symptoms worse. Consider keeping a detailed, daily record of everything you eat and drink. That way, you can more easily identify the culprit behind any prostatitis flare-ups.

Rheumatoid arthritis

Top pain-relieving remedy for stiff joints

Your body's immune system is always on the prowl for disease-causing viruses and bacteria. But sometimes your defenses get confused and attack healthy tissue. This is known as an autoimmune disease.

Rheumatoid arthritis (RA) is a condition where your body targets the lining of your joints. Rogue molecules break down the cushioning cartilage, resulting in throbbing, stiff, swollen hands, knees, or other areas. People with RA may feel tired, have occasional fevers, and generally not feel well.

You've probably tried many remedies to ease your pain, from anti-inflammatory drugs to herbal creams. You may have even tried special diets. Recent research suggests that cutting out meat and focusing on plant foods may be one of the top ways to relieve your symptoms.

"A plant-based diet comprised of fruits, vegetables, grains, and legumes may be tremendously helpful for those with rheumatoid arthritis," says Hana Kahleova, co-author of a review on plant-based diets published in *Frontiers in Nutrition*.

"This study offers hope that with a simple menu change, joint pain, swelling, and other painful symptoms may improve or even disappear," she says. So what makes this diet so powerful?

Eat	
Quinoa	Farro
Cinnamon	Turmeric
Rhubarb	Spinach
Stinging nettle	

Avoid	
Barley	Rye
Salt	Wheat

- **It fights inflammation.** Meat and fat may increase your levels of C-reactive protein (CRP), a common chemical sign of inflammation. Studies say that switching over to meals loaded with veggies, fruits, and whole grains can cause those CRP levels to plummet. Plus plant-based diets are higher in fiber, which also helps keep inflammation at bay.

- **Fiber fuels the friendly bacteria in your gut.** A healthy microbiome ferments dietary fiber into short-chain fatty acids that fight inflammation. But the trillions of good microorganisms in your gut can only do their jobs if they're part of a healthy, diverse community. Want to keep your microbiome in tiptop shape? Eat lots of fruits, vegetables, and grains.

- **Going meatless helps you shed pounds.** Carrying around a spare tire increases your risk for RA symptoms. A review of studies found that people who lost more than 11 pounds were three times more likely to relieve their joint pain compared to people who lost less than that. And a plant-based diet is one of the best ways to lose weight.

So how can you get started? You don't need to cut out meat cold turkey. Begin with a few simple meatless meals each week, like veggie stir-fries or bean chili. And try to swap out beef and chicken for other protein-heavy foods, like lentils or tofu. If you start out slow, you'll find it easier to embrace a plant-based lifestyle.

Squash RA with a heaping helping of spinach

Legend has it that when Catherine de Medici left Florence to marry into the French royal family, she brought along a host of cooks to prepare her favorite veggie — spinach. Her love of this leafy green was so great that anything served on a bed of spinach was dubbed "a la Florentine" in her honor.

But you don't need a special occasion to whip up a tasty spinach dish. It's packed with a nutrient that will help you ward off rheumatoid arthritis (RA), so you'll want to prepare it often.

Forget the pie — here's how to make the most of rhubarb

Rhubarb pie is a delicious treat, but this tart veggie can be a lot more than just a dessert. It's a powerful inflammation fighter, so a few servings can help you protect your joints. Here are two ways to add it to your table.

- Go savory by mixing it into stew or soup. Simply chop a stalk of rhubarb into 1- to 2-inch pieces, and add them to your dish to simmer during the last 15 minutes.

- Turn it into a zesty spread. Rhubarb chutney is great on meat, toast, or even in a sandwich. Add 2 tablespoons olive oil and two thinly sliced onions to a medium pot. Let them caramelize over medium heat for an hour, stirring occasionally. Then add three stalks of sliced rhubarb, a pinch of salt, and 1/2 teaspoon of sugar. Let it simmer another hour before serving.

Pile on the potassium to push back against pain. Would you believe there's a mineral that may prevent arthritis? And chances are, you don't get enough of it. But experts think that loading up on potassium could help you end needless suffering from stiffness, pain, and swelling caused by RA.

In a study published in the *American Journal of Clinical Nutrition*, researchers analyzed the diets of more than 12,500 adults and found that less than 2% of those people got enough potassium.

That's bad news — especially if you're trying to keep your joints in tiptop shape. Research shows that this nutrient is an important tool in the fight against joint pain.

In another small study, researchers tested potassium's pain-fighting prowess. They gave people with RA 6,000 milligrams (mg) of potassium chloride or a placebo every day for 28 days. At the end of the trial, the potassium group reported lower levels of pain. That's because potassium bumps up your body's levels of chemicals called glucocorticoids, which help fight inflammation.

Sup on spinach to fend off inflammation. How can you get more potassium in your diet? With your favorite leafy green, of course. A cup of cooked spinach provides you with a whopping 839 mg of this natural arthritis fighter.

Need some proof? Experts polled a group of RA sufferers to find out if the foods they ate helped — or hurt — their joints. And people singled out spinach as one of the best foods to help prevent flare-ups.

Surprise — nettle's needles soothe arthritis aches

Ever walk through a field and suddenly yelp from pain because your leg feels like it's on fire? More than likely you just walked through a patch of stinging nettle. Strange that this same plant may be just what you need to ease your rheumatoid arthritis pain.

Tiny sharp hairs on the stinging nettle plant release chemicals that irritate skin. But when you dry or cook the plant, the stinging feature goes away. Scientists have found the hairs also contain chemicals with painkilling and anti-inflammatory properties. Plus the plant is rich in vitamins and minerals.

You can use the nettle plant, powder, or dried leaves as part of your pain-relief strategy. Although research is inconclusive, the Arthritis Foundation suggests you can take up to 1,300 milligrams daily to help treat inflammation.

Look for organic nettle at specialty grocers or online. Here are some ways to use it.

- cooked as a vegetable or mixed into soups, savory dishes, pastas, and omelets
- blended as a tea or smoothie

- taken in capsule form as a supplement

- applied as a topical cream

If you take blood thinners or medication for high blood pressure, heart disease, or diabetes, ask your doctor before trying stinging nettle.

Swollen knuckles?
Skip the salt to ease your pain

A bucket of popcorn at the theater may sound like a good idea at the time, but you may regret that salty snack after the movie is over.

Three new studies suggest salt may prompt several autoimmune diseases including psoriasis, multiple sclerosis, rheumatoid arthritis, and ankylosing spondylitis, or arthritis of the spine.

Yale School of Medicine researchers discovered the link between a high-salt diet and autoimmune conditions when they conducted an animal study. They say too much salt caused the animals to produce inflammatory cells closely associated with autoimmune diseases. These cells attack healthy tissue.

To keep your sodium intake down, try to cook from scratch so you can control how much salt is in your food. If you do buy prepackaged food, look for low-sodium options.

---

2 'C's to choose when your symptoms flare

Surprising relief for your RA pain awaits — right inside your pantry. These common household spices could help take the edge off your tender, swollen joints.

Curcumin curries favor with your joints. Turmeric is all the rage in health-food circles. And for good reason, researchers say. The main chemical compound that gives turmeric its distinct golden color — curcumin — is a powerful weapon in your arsenal of anti-inflammatory foods.

A recent analysis of curcumin's effect on arthritis found that taking 1,000 milligrams of this nutrient every day for two to three months can relieve pain and swelling as well as over-the-counter drugs. To get that much from your diet, you'd need to eat about 3 1/2 tablespoons of turmeric, which could bother your stomach. Talk to your doctor about taking curcumin supplements instead.

Cinnamon helps you fight inflammation. Oatmeal, walnuts, dried cranberries, a splash of almond milk. Sounds like a wholesome breakfast. But wait. Add a dash of cinnamon, and you may help ward off the pain in your wrists when you pick up the bowl.

According to a study published in the *Journal of the American College of Nutrition*, this humble spice may relieve RA symptoms. Researchers asked a small group of women with rheumatoid arthritis to take capsules containing about 3/4 teaspoons of cinnamon or a placebo every day for eight weeks.

At the end of the study, those who ate cinnamon had lower levels of swelling, tenderness, and pain in their joints.

Put the kibosh on inflammation with ancient grains

Quinoa, sorghum, millet, amaranth, einkorn, farro, khorasan, and spelt. Chances are those unusual foods are not part of your everyday vocabulary. But they should be if you have rheumatoid arthritis.

These ancient grains are low in a group of proteins called amylase trypsin inhibitors (ATIs) that may aggravate your condition. You may be avoiding gluten to relieve your pain when actually it's ATIs you need to stay away from.

Older wheat varieties are lower in ATIs. Khorasan wheat, for example, showed anti-inflammatory results in a small trial, while modern wheat has an inflammatory effect.

By cutting foods high in ATIs, like enriched flours, wheat, barley, or rye, you may decrease inflammation and improve your RA symptoms. For more on this topic, see *Go against the grain of pain with a gluten-free diet* in the *Chronic pain* chapter.

Easy ways to slip spinach into your diet

Spinach is cheap, nutritious, and as you learned earlier in this chapter, helpful to your joints. But don't forget that spinach also tastes great. Here are some easy ways to add more spinach to your meals.

- Make salads with raw spinach. Toss with some nuts, dried fruit, cheese, and vinaigrette for added flavor and texture.

- Put spinach leaves instead of lettuce on your sandwiches.

- Saute, boil, or braise spinach to make a scrumptious side dish. Cooking spinach really concentrates the nutrients — but remember to cook more than you think you'll need, since a pound will dwindle down to about a cup after cooking.

- Spice things up. Don't like the taste of cooked spinach? Add garlic, parmesan cheese, balsamic vinegar, or nutmeg to jazz it up.

- Rethink your recipes. Add spinach to pasta dishes, casseroles, dips, soups, and egg dishes.

Sarcopenia

Recover your strength with protein

Does your staircase look as daunting as a steep mountain? Do your shoulders ache after carrying a bag of groceries? If so, you may be one of the many adults who suffer from sarcopenia, the gradual loss of muscle mass and strength.

You may not think weakening muscles are a big deal. Well, it may surprise you that sarcopenia is a leading cause of declining health as you age. It is linked to heart disease, Alzheimer's, and obesity but is entirely preventable. Although you lose about 3% of muscle mass each decade after your 30s, you'll drop even more if you don't stay active and eat right.

As you age, your body produces fewer muscle-building hormones like testosterone and the growth hormone IGF-1. Plus your body has to work even harder to convert protein and other food into energy — if you're even getting enough of it. More often than not, older adults struggle to eat a diet that provides all the nutrients they need.

Pack on the protein to pump up your muscles. You can't build a house without walls, and you can't build muscles without protein. It's the most important nutrient in your fight against sarcopenia. But there's a good chance you're not getting enough of it.

Experts think 1 out of every 5 seniors aren't eating their fill. Between decreasing appetites and changing tastes, you could be literally wasting away.

Eat

Chicken	Lentils
Tofu	Salmon
Walnuts	Beets
Spinach	Yogurt
Dark chocolate	Brazil nuts
Cheese	Fortified cereal

Avoid

Meats and grains in high quantities

How much protein do you really need? It varies based on your body type and activity level, but the general rule is 0.8 grams for every 2.2 pounds you weigh. So a 175-pound man should try to eat at least 64 grams of protein each day.

Fortunately, protein isn't too hard to come by. Half a roasted chicken breast will get you about half of your daily dose. But you don't have to limit yourself to meat protein. Research published by the *Academy of Nutrition and Dietetics* concluded that eating higher amounts of both animal and plant protein is linked with greater muscle mass. Lentils, beans, nuts, and tofu are all excellent sources of protein, too.

> Don't destroy your food's health benefits. Lentils are a great source of protein, vitamins, and minerals, but how you cook them matters. Microwaving is your best option. It's fast and easy, and won't drain away nutrients like other methods do.

Ward off sarcopenia with special supplements. As you age, you may find you lose your appetite, a circumstance called anorexia of aging. If you're not hungry, you may forget to eat, which means you're missing out on all the nutrients you need to keep you strong. The result? Muscle loss and weakness.

If you struggle with eating, talk to your doctor about adding a protein or amino acid supplement to your diet. It can help offset muscle loss that stems from inactivity and lack of nutrition. You don't have to be a bodybuilder to benefit from protein supplements. Here are three good options to consider.

- Creatine. Your liver makes enough of this protein to prevent you from becoming deficient, but adding more can help your muscles grow. It works best if you use it in addition to exercise.

- Leucine. It's an amino acid that's important in protein synthesis. Often taken with vitamin D, studies show leucine may improve muscle strength and lean mass content.

- Whey protein. This is one of the primary proteins found in dairy products. It contains leucine and other amino acids that help your muscles recover after inactivity.

Warning: Meat-heavy diets may do more harm than good

You might be tempted to load up your plate with hunks of protein-packed meats to fight off sarcopenia, but experts warn that might not be the best move. Eating too many acid-producing foods, like meat and cereal grains, can actually be bad for your body.

A buildup of acid in your tissues and blood can cause your muscles to start breaking down. In addition to making you weaker, this puts extra stress on your liver and kidneys because they have to work overtime to clean out your system.

But experts say you can keep your muscles from wasting away by eating a balanced diet that includes plenty of fruits and vegetables.

3 muscle-building nutrients keep you feeling young

Protein isn't all it takes to maintain muscle mass. But don't get intimidated by a whole slew of foods you should be eating. Keeping your muscles strong is as easy as one, two, three when you focus on this trio of nutrients.

Go fishing to stay strong — omega-3 keeps muscle loss at bay. Fish are loaded with protein, but some have another secret to staving off sarcopenia. Omega-3 fatty acids are a powerful way to fight back against waning strength.

In a recent review of 36 scientific studies, experts found that pairing omega-3 with resistance exercise is the best way to stay strong. These nutrients appear to speed up your body's natural process for building new muscle in response to strength training.

The scientists recommend that older adults get at least 1,650 milligrams each day. That may sound like a lot, but it's actually less than you'll find in a 3-ounce serving of Atlantic salmon. You can also get omega-3 from other fatty fish as well as foods like chia seeds, walnuts, and flaxseeds.

Soak up some sunshine to stay mobile and independent in your golden years. Spending all day on your couch could come back to haunt you in more ways than you think. If you stay out of the sun, you put yourself at risk for falling. New research claims low levels of vitamin D may increase your risk for muscle weakness.

A new study published in the *Journal of Physical Therapy Science* examined the vitamin D levels of 200 women over the age of 60. Researchers found that people with the lowest levels were also at the highest risk of dangerous falls.

> Scientists aren't exactly sure how vitamin D affects balance, but research has shown it has a positive action on muscles and the central nervous system. It appears to bind to a specific receptor in muscle tissue, which leads to protein synthesis and muscle cell growth.

When you're young, you don't have to worry about scanning nutrition labels for your vitamin D. Your body can make its own — all you need is a little sunlight. When ultraviolet rays hit your skin, your body starts producing this essential nutrient.

But your body does have to work harder to make vitamin D as you age, so it's a good idea to seek out vitamin D-rich foods like salmon and tuna. You can also talk to your doctor about adding supplements to your diet.

Don't "B" afraid of sarcopenia — strike back with this vital vitamin. In a recent study, scientists looked for classic signs of sarcopenia — low walking speed, grip strength, and muscle mass — in 400 older adults. The people who scored the lowest on those measurements also came up low in vitamin B12.

Scientists think vitamin B12 may play a role in preventing sarcopenia because it helps reduce blood levels of homocysteine. Studies have shown that high levels of this amino acid are related to lower muscle strength and walking speed.

The recommended daily allowance for vitamin B12 is 2.4 micrograms. It's readily available in fortified cereals, dairy, meat, and fatty fish. And if your taste runs to the unusual, good news — a single serving of liver contains 29 times your daily needs, and clams, a whopping 35.

'Beet' back sarcopenia with this surprising superfood

Believe it or not, getting up and exercising could save you $900 a year. That's how much the average person with sarcopenia shells out in health care costs. While it can be tough to get that extra bit of motivation, one food you probably never think of can help give you a little push. All it takes is a plate of beets to raise your energy level and improve your muscle function.

In a small study, scientists looked at the average time it took runners to complete a 5K — first after eating 200 grams of baked beets, which equals about 1 1/2 cups, and then again after eating cranberry relish. Surprisingly, people ran much faster after bolting down the beet meal. And even though they were running faster, people actually reported that they weren't working nearly as hard.

Scientists think the improvements in muscle performance are the result of nutrients in beets known as nitrates. These nutrients work by opening up your blood vessels to increase blood flow. This boosts oxygen delivery, powering up your muscles and taking some of the work out of your workout.

And don't worry, beets aren't the only power-packed foods. You can go for nitrate-rich options like kale, spinach, chard, or other leafy greens. However, scientists aren't quick to recommend nitrates found in processed meats like sausage and bacon. Because these foods have been linked to serious health issues, experts advise getting all your nitrates from plants.

Beet cheats to plummet prep time

Love beets or hate 'em? Everyone seems to have an opinion. But if you fall into the "hate" camp you could be missing out on a world of flavor and nutrition. Not sure what to do with them? Here's what you need to know.

- Red beets, the kind that are usually canned, have a strong earthy flavor. Fresh ones are great roasted.

- Chioggia beets are striped red and white when raw. Thinly slice them for a great salad addition.

- Golden beets are more mild than their red counterparts and don't stain. They're great raw and cooked.

Store your beets by cutting off their greens and loosely wrapping the root and greens separately. Refrigerate both parts. Leave them unwashed until you're ready to use them.

Make peeling easy by wrapping your beets in foil and roasting them for 50 to 60 minutes at 450 degrees. When they cool, use a paper towel to slip the skin right off.

Enlist these mighty minerals to maintain your muscle mass

It's easy to get wrapped up in calories, fats, and vitamins when you're reading a nutrition label, but you need to make sure you're not missing one important little section tucked at the bottom —

the minerals. These essential nutrients could be the difference between staying in your own house and ending up in a nursing home. Check out three muscle-savers that can aid in your fight against sarcopenia.

Maximize your might with magnesium. Did you know one of your best bets for preventing muscle loss is found in delicious dark chocolate? In a recent study published in *Nutrients*, researchers looked at more than 156,000 men and women and found that eating more magnesium-packed foods was associated with better grip strength and muscle mass.

How does it work? Scientists think magnesium plays a vital role in muscle function and performance. Plus the nutrient is involved in building and repairing your muscles.

Experts say men should try to get 420 milligrams (mg) of magnesium every day, and women, 320 mg. Mix up your menu by eating high-magnesium foods like dark chocolate, almonds, and cooked spinach.

Seek out selenium to stay strong. Want to rev up muscle power? Make sure you get enough selenium. Researchers think this mineral helps your body create substances called selenoprotiens, which work to build and maintain strong, healthy muscles.

In a recent review, scientists examined 10 studies that looked at the link between diet and muscle size and strength in folks over 64. Experts found that people who didn't eat much selenium were much more likely to suffer from sarcopenia.

But getting this nutrient doesn't need to be difficult — a single Brazil nut contains a little bit more than your entire recommended daily dose. You can also find it in cod, tuna, and sunflower seeds. Just shoot for 55 micrograms of selenium every day.

Cut sarcopenia risk by chowing down on calcium. Vitamin D deficiencies often go hand in hand with calcium shortages, so some people blame the sunshine vitamin without giving calcium a second thought. But the latest research says skimping on calcium can eat away at your muscles, even if you get enough vitamin D.

More studies are needed to work out how calcium helps build muscles, but for now make sure you get at least 1,200 mg each day. Step up your calcium game with foods like mozzarella cheese, yogurt, and sardines.

The surprising connection between your mouth and muscles

By now you know that what you eat can drastically affect how well you maintain muscle as you age. What you may not realize is your mouth plays a bigger role than you think. Here's why.

- If you have poor oral health, you may start limiting your diet choices. Avoiding hard foods like meats, fruits, and vegetables could seem like the safest option. But that means you're missing out on rich sources of protein, vitamins, and other nutrients, raising your risk for malnutrition and frailty. Mix more fruits and veggies into your diet to improve your oral health with natural antioxidant power. And don't forget to brush and floss to keep your teeth and gums strong.

- The muscles in your jaw are affected by sarcopenia too, and as they weaken you may have difficulty chewing and swallowing. If that happens, getting the nutrients you lack could be as simple as preparing foods differently. Try mincing or pureeing meats and vegetables to make them easier to eat.

Eat better than the Queen to safeguard your strength

England's Queen Elizabeth II has enjoyed a surprisingly long reign considering her country's standard diet is thought to be one of the worst for your health.

Traditional British fare includes red meat, potatoes, gravy, and butter. Although Brits may see them as comfort foods, having a large proportion of them in your meals may increase your risk of sarcopenia.

Protein is a big factor in fending off weak muscles, but alone it's not enough. You need to look at your diet as a whole rather than just at a few nutrients.

Upgrade your food choices to stave off sarcopenia. Foodies across the pond aren't the only ones who are at risk because of their eating habits. American studies have also linked poor diet to sarcopenia.

In a recent study published by the *Journal of the American Geriatrics Society*, 2,154 older Americans were followed for four years to chart their diet and frailty. Signs of being frail included a weak hand grip, regularly feeling exhausted, walking slowly, and losing more than 5% of body weight over the previous year.

- Participants with poor-quality diets were almost twice as likely to become frail as those with high-quality diets. And even those who ate a medium-quality diet had a 40% higher risk of frailty.

- The best diets scored high on the healthy eating index, which means they followed government dietary recommendations like the Food Guide Pyramid. High-quality diets include more beneficial foods like fruits, vegetables, and fish, and fewer nutrient-poor foods like refined grains and sweets.

Manage your microbiome for muscle protection. Your food choices help determine whether you have good or bad bacteria living in your digestive tract. And your gut can influence functions throughout your entire body. That's why an unhealthy microbiome may play such a big role in sarcopenia.

One of the causes of sarcopenia is inflammation. As you age, you lose diversity in your microbiome and tend to create more bad bacteria. That change may increase the inflammation level in your body and contribute to muscle loss.

Ramp up the power of your microbiome by eating foods like wild salmon, kimchi and other fermented foods, and nonstarchy fruits and vegetables like tomatoes, carrots, cherries, and grapefruit. These foods are rich in beneficial bacteria and fiber that are essential for a healthy gut.

Don't limit yourself to eating right, though. Physical activity is also good for your muscles — and your microbiome. Research has shown that both your exercise routine and food choices can improve your gut's diversity.

Sinusitis

Don't let a low vitamin D level fuel your congestion

Your sinuses are a connected system of hollow cavities behind your nose, cheeks, and lower forehead. When everything is running smoothly, you hardly think of them. But when something goes wrong, like sinusitis, boy, do you notice.

Sinusitis is really just inflammation of your sinuses and nasal passages. The membrane lining your sinuses produces mucus, which normally flows out through your nose. When something irritates that membrane, like a cold virus, allergies, cigarette smoke, or bacteria, it swells. The swelling blocks the exit route to your nose, trapping air and mucus in your sinuses. As the mucus gets thicker, bacteria may start to flourish, setting the stage for a secondary infection.

Doctors classify sinusitis by how long it lasts — acute lasts fewer than four weeks, subacute between four and 12 weeks, and chronic more than 12 weeks. If you have more than three episodes in one year, you have recurrent sinusitis.

You can ease your symptoms with lifestyle approaches like nasal irrigation or an array of medications. Some even go the route of sinus surgery if symptoms persist. But eating to lower inflammation may be your best dietary strategy because constant inflammation leads to diseases like chronic rhinosinusitis (CRS), another name for chronic sinusitis.

As you get older, your immune and inflammatory responses change. With CRS, researchers suggest the change could mean corticosteroid

Eat	
Cheese	Tuna
Eggs	Oysters
Pork	Beef liver
UV-exposed mushrooms	
D-fortified tofu	

Avoid

High-sugar foods like doughnuts and soda

medications that once provided relief no longer seem to have an effect. So it's even more important to prevent a recurrence if you can. New research points to one natural way of doing that.

Get the lowdown on low D. Vitamin D has already proven itself to be a superstar nutrient in the *Asthma* and *Colds & Flu* chapters. So it's really no surprise that the latest studies say it may do wonders for your sinuses, too.

Low levels of vitamin D — particularly D3, the kind found in animal-based foods — puts you at risk for allergic diseases like CRS. In fact, a recent meta-analysis of eight studies confirmed that low levels are associated with chronic sinusitis.

Getting enough D is important because it helps block inflammation and support your immune response. That's why researchers say supplementing with vitamin D may help people with CRS.

Drop more D onto your plate. It's not as hard as you might think to increase your vitamin D through food. Try adding D-rich foods like oysters, fortified tofu, UV-exposed portobello mushrooms, egg yolks, cheese, pork spareribs, beef liver, or canned tuna to your menu during the week.

Wondering how to work these into your regular menu? Ask yourself how your local diner might do it. Their menu might look something like this.

- baked oysters with mushroom ragout

- classic beef liver and onions

- Chinese steamed pork spareribs and tofu

- tuna salad with chopped egg

- three cheese stuffed mushrooms

- tuna mushroom casserole

Shed some light on your mushrooms

Mushrooms make vitamin D when they bask in UV rays. Unfortunately, commercially produced varieties generally get raised in the dark, then quickly picked under a fluorescent light. Chances are they're not meeting your vitamin D needs. But you can fix that say researchers who tested these methods on fresh button mushrooms.

- Slice your mushrooms, lay them out flat on a pan, and expose them to midday sunlight for 15 to 120 minutes. They'll make enough vitamin D per serving to meet half the daily recommended amount or more.

- Refrigerate your sunlight-exposed mushrooms and use them within a week. Their vitamin D levels may start to wane after eight days, on average.

- Boil UV-exposed button mushrooms for 20 minutes or bake them for 10 minutes and you'll hold on to up to 67% of their D. Pan-fry them five minutes to keep more of their D — up to 88%.

Tame inflammation with a bromelain boost

Did you know a pineapple plant can only make one pineapple at a time, and it will take twice as long as it takes a woman to have a child? No wonder it's got so much therapeutic potential.

Pineapples contain an enzyme called bromelain, which you can get as a supplement. It's impressing the socks off researchers for its possible health benefits with bronchitis, arthritis, wound healing, and even cancer. And it may be the remedy you've been looking for to control sinusitis inflammation.

Researchers say it may work on inflammation in two ways — first to activate a healthy immune reaction, and second to calm down an overactive immune response. That could be why early studies showed it improved symptom scores in folks with chronic sinusitis.

How much should you take? In one recent small study, researchers gave participants with chronic sinusitis a 500-milligram bromelain tablet twice a day for one month. Afterward they found high concentrations of the nutrient in the participants' nasal cells, a strong indicator of its protective potential in upper airways. You can get the same 30-day supply for under $10 at your local pharmacy.

If you're taking blood thinner medication, you should not take bromelain. Check with your doctor to see if a bromelain supplement could treat your sinusitis.

Control your sweet tooth to fight sinusitis

Want to cripple your sinus defenses? Go ahead and eat that doughnut. Sweets are a surefire way to shift the balance of power to the bacterial invaders in your sinuses. Here's why you should step away from the sugar if you're prone to sinusitis.

Let your taste buds do their job. Your taste buds — and even other parts of your body like your upper airway and digestive tract — are armed with bitter and sweet taste receptors, though only those in your mouth send the taste sensation to your brain. The bitter receptors are standing guard for your sinuses against bacteria and fungi that seek to do you harm.

When certain bacteria and fungi make their way into your airway, they give off a compound your bitter taste receptors may pick up. Your receptors then set off an alarm in your immune system. The message to fight the bad guys goes out within seconds to minutes.

Unfortunately, the sweet taste receptors don't see the world as a hostile place. They welcome bacteria and tell their bitter counterparts to sit back and relax. In other words, when you trigger your sweet taste receptors, you're telling those defensive bitter taste receptors to be quiet.

Don't excite your sweet tooth. The sweet taste receptors mean well. But what they're really doing when they get excited is allowing the bad guys past your built-in alarm system. Researchers already know that some bacteria use this to their advantage.

Staphylococcus aureus, which has been linked to sinusitis and other diseases caused by upper airway inflammation, is one such beast. Scientists discovered it can produce amino acids associated with sweetness at a concentration high enough to hold back your body's normal immune response to bitter taste receptors.

So what's a body to do? Well, researchers have already shown that eating lots of sugar may be linked to inflammatory stress and sinus symptoms. So pass on the sweet potato casserole and indulge in some oven-roasted Brussels sprouts instead. Your nose will thank you.

Deflate swollen sinuses with new herbal concoctions

Ever heard of phytoneering? It's a process where scientists engineer better natural medicines by identifying powerful ingredients and combining herbal extracts. The results are promising.

In one study, for example, participants with acute bacterial sinusitis took a phytoneering herbal supplement in addition to their regular antibiotic and decongestant treatment. The herbs included cowslip, gentian, common sorrel, elder, and vervain. They reported greater improvements in symptoms like swelling, stuffy nose, and headache than the control group.

Although it's still too early for a solid recommendation, experts suggest the phytoneering supplement, sold under the name Sinupret, may enhance standard therapy.

Skin cancer

Body of proof: Some fatty foods can raise skin cancer risk

Remember high school summers spent soaking up the sun? You slathered yourself with baby oil and iodine, hoping to achieve a deep golden tan. But, oh the damage you did to your skin. So what can you do now to keep from paying a heavy price for your sun-worshipping teenage years?

Understand what you need to look for. Experts say too much exposure to the sun's ultraviolet (UV) light is the main cause of most skin cancers. Why? The UV rays can damage the DNA in your skin cells and cause them to multiply uncontrollably. Look out for these three major types of skin cancer.

- Basal cell carcinoma (BCC) is the most common form of skin cancer, with more than 4 million cases diagnosed in the U.S. annually. BCC often crops up as red patches, pearly bumps, or scar-like lesions on your face, neck, scalp, or shoulders.

- Squamous cell carcinoma (SCC) often surfaces on your scalp, hands, ears, or lips. But these flat, crusty lesions can also appear in your mouth or on the soles of your feet. SCC can grow deep into the layers of your skin and spread to other parts of the body.

- Melanoma typically develops as a spot on the skin or a change in the shape, size, or color of an existing mole. In men, it most often develops on the chest and back. Women tend to get melanoma on their arms and legs. Along with UV rays, genetics may cause the disease to develop.

Eat	
Apricots	Tomato paste
Red grapes	Tuna
Blueberries	Olive oil
Dark chocolate	

Avoid
Safflower oil and corn oil
Heavily processed foods

When in doubt, check it out. The best way to reduce your risk of skin cancer is by making good lifestyle choices, like limiting your time in the sun. And using sunscreen is essential. But you'll still want to monitor your skin for worrisome changes.

That's because 99% of all cases are curable if treated early enough. So take a few minutes to examine your skin each month. See your doctor right away if you find anything suspicious.

But what about other ways to protect yourself? Surprise! The answer could be in the foods you eat.

Studies suggest that resveratrol — a polyphenol found in red grapes, dark chocolate, peanuts, and blueberries — slows the growth of skin cancer cells. But your gut breaks down resveratrol very quickly, so it doesn't stay in your system long enough to do much good. That's why scientists are developing topical creams with more staying power.

Protect the skin you're in. Researchers have found that polyunsaturated fats — especially the omega-6 fatty acids that your body uses for energy — may increase your risk of skin cancer. Studies suggest high amounts of omega-6 boost production of prostaglandin E, a hormone-like compound associated with inflammation and cancer.

Experts say men should eat no more than 14 grams of omega-6 a day. That drops to 11 grams for women. But with omega-6 fatty acids hiding in lots of your favorite foods, it's easy to go overboard. A tablespoon of mayonnaise made with safflower or soybean oil, for example, has a whopping 7 grams.

Your best bet? Check food labels before loading up your shopping cart. Switch from using corn oil, which is high in omega-6 fatty acids, for a more healthy olive oil. And remember that most heavily processed foods — think chicken nuggets, french fries, cookies, crackers, and sweets — are made with oils packed with omega-6.

Tomato's powerful lycopene cans cancer cells

How do you fix a broken tomato? With tomato paste, of course. A silly joke, to be sure, but there's interesting science behind it. For example, researchers believe a compound in tomatoes called lycopene may shield your skin from the sun's damaging rays.

Does that mean tomato paste could protect you from skin cancer? You might be surprised.

Scientists tested the idea in a small study of women who sunburned easily. Half the participants added a little more than 3 tablespoons of tomato paste — that's 16 milligrams of lycopene — to their diet every day for 12 weeks. The other half didn't. Three months later, tests on the volunteers who ate the tomato paste showed that their skin's protection against ultraviolet rays improved by 30%.

Of course tomatoes are no substitute for a good sunscreen. But the next time you're enjoying some pasta, add a little tomato sauce — for your skin's sake.

Bag a laundry list of benefits from apricots

Want to live a longer life? There's an "ap" for that. That's right. "Ap" — as in apricot. This little Turkish delight has been around for centuries, pleasing palates all over the world. But it has only recently come into its own as a crowd-pleasing superfood.

Turns out people who eat apricots may not only avoid skin cancer, but also heart disease, high blood pressure, high cholesterol, and Alzheimer's disease. They might even live longer. Take your pick — enjoy apricots fresh, dried, or canned.

A study of the dietary habits of nearly 124,000 adults over more than two decades found that those with the highest average daily intake of vitamin A were 17% less likely to develop squamous cell carcinoma (SCC) than those with the least amount. Researchers believe retinoids — compounds found in abundance in vitamin A — prevent cancer cells from multiplying.

"Skin cancer, including squamous cell carcinoma, is hard to prevent, but this study suggests that eating a healthy diet rich in vitamin A may be a way to reduce your risk, in addition to wearing sunscreen and reducing sun exposure," says Eunyoung Cho, associate professor of dermatology and epidemiology at Brown University.

More research is needed to find out how much vitamin A you need to lower your SCC risk. But experts recommend that men get 900 micrograms (mcg) each day. Just 10 dried apricot halves provide 25% of that amount. Women should get 700 mcg a day.

Choose a 'cot a Marine would love

Oh, apricots. Astronauts love 'em. In fact, they were among the first snacks eaten on the moon. But the Marines won't touch 'em. Tradition holds they bring bad luck. Read on for tips to help you pick and prepare this delicious fruit. Who knows? You might even win over a Marine.

Ripe apricots have a rich, orange color and are slightly soft to the touch. If you pick one that's yellow or green, allow it to ripen in a closed paper bag at room temperature for three to four days. You can refrigerate ripe apricots in a plastic bag for a day or two.

Wash the fruit under running water before eating. Carefully cut around the apricot's seam with a paring knife, twist the fruit into halves, and pull out the pit. Enjoy your apricot right away, or brush its cut surfaces with lemon juice so they don't turn brown.

Stress & Anxiety

Burnout Rx: A sweet treat keeps you on your feet

You've just won a prize. In the midst of cheers and applause, everyone in the room turns to congratulate you. Your palms go clammy, your shoulders tense, and you feel unsteady on your feet. What's happening?

Your body is responding to stress, albeit the good kind. The physical changes you experience — a racing heart, fast-paced breathing, and increased blood pressure — are normal, temporary reactions. But if stress weighs on you for long periods, your health could suffer.

Know that stress can creep up on you. Ever get into a really scary situation? If so, your adrenal glands released adrenaline and cortisol, hormones that sound an alarm readying you for a fight-or-flight response. Most likely, your hormone levels returned to normal once the threat was gone.

But sometimes that doesn't happen. Say, for example, you're caring for a sick loved one or having trouble paying the bills. The constant worry means your body is overexposed to stress hormones, putting you at risk for a host of health problems.

Oddly enough, you may not even realize you're under emotional strain. But your body does. You may be gaining weight and having trouble sleeping and not even realize the cause. Not many people know it, but stress is a secret cause of excess belly fat, sleeplessness, and high blood pressure.

Fortunately, you can learn to relax even when under pressure. Experts recommend activities like

Eat

Anchovies	Chia seeds
Tempeh	Holy basil tea
Mackerel	Matcha green tea
Saffron	Dark chocolate
Salmon	Sauerkraut

Avoid

Highly processed food

dancing, singing, laughing, and even crying. Making time for hobbies and relaxation also helps. But treating yourself to dark chocolate?

Dark chocolate brings sweet relief. Novel writer Geraldine Solon says, "When things are rough all you need is chocolate." The award-winning author must have done her homework. Scientists say eating dark chocolate may be an amazingly easy, no-drug solution to relieving stress.

In a month-long study, researchers found that participants who ate 3/4 ounce of dark chocolate with 65.7% cocoa solids and 2% total flavonoids every day had significantly lower cortisol levels than volunteers who ate the same amount of dark chocolate with 56% cocoa solids and only tiny traces of the phytonutrient. The scientists believe flavonoids prevent an enzyme from converting cortisone into the stress hormone cortisol.

But set yourself limits. Dark chocolate contains sugar and fat, so moderation is best.

How to get fast relief from stress and mental fatigue

British civilians during World War II turned to a popular herb to cope with the constant threat of air raids. It was valerian, a plant that's been used for hundreds of years to relieve tension.

New research suggests this popular extract might be just what you need to give your brain a boost. Scientists gave 64 volunteers who reported feeling psychologically stressed 100 milligrams of valerian root extract or a placebo three times a day for four weeks. Participants interviewed with a psychiatrist and had their brain waves tested at the beginning and end of the study.

Surprisingly, both groups showed improvements in their anxiety and other psychiatric symptoms. But things got interesting when the researchers tested the participants' brain waves. They found significant increases in the valerian group's alpha wave activity.

Your brain produces alpha waves when you're awake but feeling relaxed, like when you're daydreaming or falling asleep.

That wasn't the whole story, though. The valerian group also saw decreases in their theta wave activity. Some studies link strong theta wave activity with anxiety and negative thoughts or emotions. The researchers say valerian may have helped the volunteers process their feelings better.

Hungry and tired? Think twice before turning to a quick fix like frozen pizza. Highly processed foods can cause sugar and insulin imbalances that increase anxiety levels. A diet full of whole grains, fruits, and veggies is a healthier option that will also improve your ability to deal with stress.

How can one little plant alter your brain's electrical activity? Scientists believe valerian contains natural compounds that help your nerve cells release a chemical called gamma-aminobutyric acid, or GABA. When GABA attaches to a protein in your brain — dubbed the GABA receptor — it relaxes you, making you feel less stressed and anxious.

You can find valerian in the supplement aisle at most pharmacies. Be sure to check with your doctor to see if valerian interacts with any medications you're taking.

Probiotics power — it's time to go with your gut

An axis can be a powerful thing. Take the earth, for example. It rotates around this center line every 24 hours to give you sunny days and starry nights. Your body, meanwhile, has a gut-brain axis — a communication system between your central nervous system and the trillions of microorganisms in your intestinal tract — that plays a big role in your emotional state.

So if you're suffering from stress or anxiety, you might just need to tweak your gut bacteria to get back on track.

Change the gut-brain conversation. Ever feel nauseated before a big test? It's no wonder considering how your brain can make you feel as if you've got butterflies in your stomach. It turns out, though, that the connection goes both ways.

Research suggests that flora in your intestines can affect your brain. In fact, studies suggest the right kind of gut bacteria might boost your mood and even combat anxiety and depression. Conversely, the wrong kind may do the opposite.

Perk up with probiotics. Probiotics — live bacteria and yeast that are good for you — may be just what the doctor ordered when it comes to boosting your mood. A review of 14 studies of people who used probiotics to regulate their intestinal bacteria found that 36% of them found supplements helped reduce anxiety symptoms like irritability, dry mouth, and restlessness.

Researchers say all of the participants took one or more of the following bacterial strands — *Lactobacillus*, *Streptococcus*, and *Bifidobacterium*. The scientists say more investigation is needed to explain the results, but other research suggests certain probiotics secrete chemicals that influence your mood.

Get your fill with these fine foods. Why take supplements when you can enjoy super healthy probiotic foods? Fortunately, you can find pretty much all you need at the supermarket. Fermented foods like yogurt, sauerkraut, tempeh, and some kinds of cheese are teeming with good bacteria.

Get your fill of *Lactobacillus*, say, by adding sauerkraut to your diet. Raw, fermented cabbage adds a zing to salads, sandwiches, and even scrambled eggs. You can also toss tempeh — a soy-based product with a nutty flavor — into tacos to help your *Bifidobacterium* thrive.

Eat happy — fruits and veggies to the rescue

What might happen if you spent less time biting your nails from stress and more time nibbling on fruits and vegetables? You'd have great looking fingernails. You might also feel less tense and edgy.

Fret less with fruits and veggies. People who stick to plant-based foods report being less stressed and anxious than those who include meat in their diets. Some suspect it's because they're not getting an omega-6 polyunsaturated fatty acid commonly found in poultry, seafood, and meat.

So what's so bad about this compound called arachidonic acid? While it has health benefits, it's also an inflammatory that has been linked to depression and other mental health issues.

Little shifts bring big results. Sliced or diced, just eating fruits and veggies more often can improve your outlook on life. That's according to data taken over seven years on 45,000 people in the United Kingdom. Researchers found that increasing the amount of fruit and veggies eaten by just one serving a day improved the participants' mental well-being. How much in a serving? A cup of raw vegetables, half a cup of cooked vegetables or fruit, or a single piece of fruit.

The federal government recommends you eat at least 1 1/2 to 2 cups of fruit and 2 to 3 cups of vegetables each day. Here's what else studies suggest fruits and veggies might do for you.

- lower levels of depression, anxiety, and fear
- maintain healthy cells
- increase levels of the hormone serotonin in your brain
- make it less likely that you'll eat unhealthy foods

Start fishing for a solution to anxiety

How do you react when fearful and uneasy? When the batfish gets scared, it floats on its side and looks like a fallen mangrove leaf drifting along the water's surface. Happily, you don't have to take such extreme measures when stress comes a knocking.

Just make sure you get enough omega-3 polyunsaturated fatty acids (PUFAs). A recent analysis of years of research found that a lack of omega-3 PUFAs in your diet can increase your chances of becoming depressed and anxious.

So what's one of the fatty acids that plays an important role in your brain health? Docosahexaenoic acid (DHA). This important fat helps the mood-boosting chemical serotonin transmit information between nerve cells. Research has also linked low levels of DHA in the blood with high levels of cortisol — your body's stress hormone.

It's easy to increase the amount of omega-3 PUFAs you eat. Load up on fatty fish like salmon, mackerel, herring, sardines, and anchovies on a regular basis. Ground flaxseed, chia seeds, walnuts, and canola oil are also excellent sources.

Have a spot of tea to calm down

Does a glass of iced tea help you relax? You may be interested in learning that the drink was created from a stressful situation at the 1904 St. Louis World's Fair. The weather was so stifling that a hot tea merchant couldn't even give away his samples. So he grabbed ice from a neighboring vendor, dropped it into his tea, and voila — an American tradition was born.

Today, tea — whether cold or hot — is a mainstay for calming frayed nerves and clearing your head. Many teas will help you relax, but two in particular are known for their stress-fighting prowess.

Matcha says "gotcha" to tension. Ever hear of matcha tea? The key ingredient to Japanese tea ceremonies for centuries, matcha is a green tea that is ground into a fine powder and whisked into hot water before serving.

Among all teas, matcha is said to have the highest concentration of L-theanine. That's important because research suggests this amino acid sparks alpha brain wave activity — the kind that occurs when you're relaxed. It also raises levels of dopamine, a "feel-good" chemical that carries messages between brain cells.

Researchers say only high-quality matcha relieves anxiety. They found that just 42% of the matcha marketed in Japan had the correct balance of compounds — including L-theanine — to tackle stress. Learn to pick the right matcha in *Looking for relief? Make the right matcha choice.*

Holy basil soothes the spirit. The Hindi name for this powerful herb is tulsi — the incomparable one. It's easy to see why. Holy basil has been used in traditional Indian medicine for centuries, treating conditions ranging from hiccups and rheumatism to heart disease and asthma.

It looks like holy basil does even more. A review of several studies of people who took the herb found it significantly lowered their stress-related symptoms. You can find holy basil tea — it has a pepper flavor with a note of clove — at your local supermarket.

But this herb isn't for everyone. Holy basil may increase your chances of bruising and bleeding if you're taking blood thinners like heparin, warfarin, and aspirin.

Rally your mood with saffron — the sunshine spice

You've probably heard how outrageously expensive saffron can be. A single pound of this sweetly floral spice can run thousands of dollars.

That's because crocus growers must tediously pluck — by hand — the three, threadlike stigmas from a single flower to get just the tiniest bit of saffron. In fact, you'd need 70,000 crocus blossoms to collect a pound of the orange-yellow spice. But if you're anxious, saffron could be worth its weight in gold.

A recent review of several studies found that people who took saffron supplements experienced a significant reduction in anxiety symptoms compared with those who took placebos. Researchers believe the results may be due to saffron's antioxidant and anti-inflammatory properties.

Many supermarkets sell saffron supplements. Or you could buy the real deal. But remember that a little bit goes a long way. Just a few threads of saffron will add a subtle flavor and aroma — and a golden hue — to your stews, rice, and seafood dishes.

Looking for relief?
Make the right matcha choice

So you heard matcha green tea has a calming effect. But when you search for it online, all the confusing options just get you hot under the collar. Here's how to easily recognize the best matcha for you.

Most importantly, you'll want to avoid buying matcha with even a hint of bitterness. A lack of sweetness indicates the tea contains compounds that can reduce its stress-reducing effects.

Which is why you'll want to look for matcha that has any of these words on its packaging.

- sweet or umami

- tender leaves

- gyokuro or ichibancha

- ceremonial grade

Because matcha comes in a powder, you'll need to sift 1 to 2 teaspoons into a cup before adding hot water. Whisk vigorously until the tea is frothy. Serve and enjoy.

Stroke

Mind your minerals: Key to a healthy head and heart

Way back in 1987, you may have heard a collective sigh of relief. That's when news broke that you could reduce your chance of having a deadly stroke up to a whopping 40% simply by adding more foods with potassium to your meals. Strokes continue to be debilitating or deadly, and preventing them is a top priority.

A stroke is an interruption in blood flow to your brain. An ischemic stroke, the most common type, happens when an artery supplying the brain gets blocked. On the other hand, if a blood vessel tears and bleeds into the brain, it's called a hemorrhagic stroke.

Balance these minerals to get the golden ratio for heart health. It's no stroke of luck. Evidence from the Multi-Ethnic Study of Atherosclerosis (MESA) in older adults shows that having higher levels of potassium than sodium in your urine — or even the same amount of both — is linked to a 40% to 50% lower risk of stroke.

Dietary guidelines recommend you aim for at least 4,700 milligrams (mg) of potassium and less than 2,300 mg of sodium each day. What researchers have found for many years, though, is Americans often get more sodium than they do potassium — the opposite of what the recommendations say.

What do experts suggest to improve heart health? Pump up potassium and lower sodium by eating a diet high in fruits, vegetables, fish, nuts, whole grains, and dairy.

Eat

Almonds	Apples
Bananas	Cocoa
Collard greens	Beans
Milk	Peanut butter
Pears	Swiss chard
Yams	Yogurt

Avoid

Foods high in sodium

Artificially sweetened drinks

Put some prevention on your plate. A meta-analysis of 16 studies involving 639,440 participants published in the *Journal of the American Heart Association* had promising results. They found that getting about 3,500 milligrams of potassium a day was associated with the lowest risk of stroke.

Eating that much throughout the day is easy.

- Add a small box of raisins (322 mg) to a cup of low-fat yogurt (531 mg) at breakfast. Chase it with a cup of orange juice (496 mg).

- Snack on a large wedge of cantaloupe (272 mg).

- Lunch on a half cup of lima beans (478 mg) alongside 3 ounces of halibut (449 mg) served over a cup of quinoa (318 mg).

- Make your afternoon snack an ounce of unsalted roasted almonds (209 mg).

- For dinner, serve up a half cup each of cooked yams (456 mg) and Great Northern beans (460 mg), and a cup of cooked Swiss chard (961 mg).

And voila, 4,952 mg of potassium — just over your daily goal.

Clean up your arteries with collards

You don't have to wait until New Year's Day to whip up a traditional batch of collard greens for good luck. You can keep your arteries clear and beat the odds of having a stroke by eating this delicious down-home vegetable all year long.

Green leafy vegetables like collards are rich in nitrates, phytochemicals, flavonoids, polyphenols, and omega-3 fatty acids. These may play a role in reducing oxidative stress, inflammation, and blood pressure — all of which have major impacts on the health of your blood vessels.

Check out two ways collards clean house in your arteries.

Powerful vitamins that neutralize artery-clogging toxins. One study found that men who got more folate and vitamin B6 in their diets were less likely to die from heart failure. Women who ate more folate and B6 were less likely to die from stroke and heart disease.

Why? These B vitamins help your body convert and use homocysteine, an amino acid that is both produced in your body and found in meat. This process lowers the amount of homocysteine in your bloodstream. That's good, because too much artery-damaging homocysteine circulating in your blood puts you at risk for heart disease.

So get a pot of collards cooking, because 1 cup delivers about 12% of your daily recommended amount of B6 and 44% of your daily folate.

> When it comes to recognizing a stroke, experts want you to BE FAST. Pay attention to Balance, Eyes, Face, Arms, Speech, and Time. If you suddenly have trouble with coordination, blurred vision, numbness or weakness in your face or arms, or slurred speech, you should seek medical care immediately.

Vitamin C clobbers cholesterol. This impressive vitamin uses its antioxidant powers to stop LDL oxidation, which happens when LDL cholesterol is damaged by chemical interactions with free radicals. Oxidized LDL can cause hardened arteries, increasing your chances of heart attack or stroke.

In a study of 82,044 Japanese men and women, nonsmokers who got the most vitamin C from their food were less likely to have a stroke. Collards happen to be rich in vitamin C — 1 cup has 38% of the recommended amount for men and 46% for women.

What's the best way to cook them? Steaming your collards improves their ability to bind bile acids, which helps your body get rid of cholesterol. To learn the easiest way to steam your greens, read the box *Give grandma's collards a healthier twist* in the chapter *Age-related macular degeneration*.

Protein perks — the right balance guards blood vessels

Did you know an ounce of roasted crickets has 2 1/2 times more protein than an ounce of beef? Not that you'd want to serve up insects for dinner, but you should think about how you're getting protein in your diet. Why? This nutrient may keep you merry as a cricket by protecting you from a stroke.

Deliver a protein punch to prevent stroke. Researchers recently discovered that the more protein you eat, the better your chances of dodging a stroke. In their study of 2,400 Japanese men and women age 40 to 79 over a 19-year period, they concluded that the protective effect on blood vessels may be due to nonessential amino acids, the building blocks of proteins.

- The risk of total and ischemic stroke dropped 40% for those eating more vegetable protein compared to those who ate the least. Researchers say nonessential amino acids like arginine may have contributed by lowering blood pressure and improving glucose tolerance.

- Compared to those who ate the least animal protein, participants who ate the most had a 53% lower risk of intracerebral hemorrhage, a type of hemorrhagic stroke that causes bleeding in brain tissue. An earlier study suggested cysteine, a nonessential amino acid in eggs, poultry, and whole grains, may play a role in lowering stroke risk by reducing oxidative stress.

Balance protein sources by veering toward veggies. Is any one protein source better than the other? Well, a recent study on middle-aged adults says plant foods may take the prize.

"While you don't have to give up foods derived from animals completely, our study does suggest that eating a larger proportion of plant-based foods and a smaller proportion of animal-based foods may help reduce your risk of having a heart attack, stroke, or other type of cardiovascular disease," says lead researcher,

Casey M. Rebholz, Ph.D., assistant professor of epidemiology at Johns Hopkins Bloomberg School of Public Health.

"To reduce cardiovascular disease risk people should eat more vegetables, nuts, whole grains, fruits, legumes and fewer animal-based foods," she says. "These findings are pretty consistent with previous findings about other dietary patterns, including the Dietary Approaches to Stop Hypertension, or DASH diet, which emphasize the same food items."

Look for the plant protein powerhouses. Wondering which vegetables are the heavy lifters when it comes to protein? Check out the legume family — edamame, lentils, chickpeas, pinto beans. Or pick up a handful of mixed nuts with some pistachios, almonds, and peanuts.

Diet drinks pose stroke danger for women

Artificial sweeteners range from 200 to 20,000 times sweeter than table sugar. Lots of folks swear by them for weight control, but a study just published by the American Heart Association in the journal *Stroke* found a higher risk of ischemic stroke in women who drink artificially sweetened beverages (ASB). Here's what you should know.

The study followed 81,714 postmenopausal women age 50 to 79 for an average of nearly 12 years as they participated in the Women's Health Initiative Observational Study. Those who drank two or more ASBs a day had a 23% higher stroke risk compared to those who drank less than once a week or never.

They were especially prone to small artery occlusion strokes, a type of ischemic stroke caused by blockage of one of the small arteries in the brain. This research leads some experts to think the process by which blood vessels get damaged may differ for ischemic and hemorrhagic strokes.

Stroke of genius has researchers backing white fruits

It's amazing what you can learn from a math model. That's how researchers estimated that by eating more of just one fruit, Americans could avoid 8,500 heart attacks and strokes each year and stave off diabetes.

All things being equal, pick the apple. That's right, in a clever test of the famous expression "an apple a day keeps the doctor away," experts collected data on the hypothetical scenario of prescribing either a daily apple or cholesterol-lowering statin drug to every person over 50 years old in the United Kingdom. What they found might surprise you.

Assuming 70% of the population followed instructions, the calculations revealed that prescribing an apple a day or a statin a day would likely have the same effect of preventing stroke. The trade-off is that statins can lead to muscle diseases and diabetes.

> Studies show that getting more dairy may lower your stroke risk. But that doesn't mean you have to stick to boring ol' milk. Fermented dairy, in particular, is also linked to a lower risk — maybe because it is tied to lower levels of artery-plugging LDL cholesterol. Jazz up your snack time with yogurt, kefir, ricotta cheese, cottage cheese, or sour cream.

If you're already taking statins, you shouldn't replace them with apples. But if you're trying to prevent blood vessel trouble without potential side effects, adding more of the flavorful fruit could have its benefits.

Make way for more light-colored treats. White-fleshed fruits, like apples and pears, are deliciously rich sources of flavonoids and fiber.

- Flavonoids are known to lower bad cholesterol and raise good cholesterol, among many other anti-inflammatory benefits.

- Pectin — the main soluble fiber found in apples and pears — helps transport and absorb nutrients, sugars, and fats in your body. Experts believe it lowers cholesterol which may combat the plaque buildup in your arteries that leads to blockages and stroke.

One 10-year study of 20,069 people found the risk of stroke was 52% lower for those who ate higher numbers of white fruits and vegetables compared those who ate lower numbers.

"To prevent stroke, it may be useful to consume considerable amounts of white fruits and vegetables," said Linda M. Oude Griep, M.Sc., lead author of the study and a postdoctoral fellow in human nutrition at Wageningen University in the Netherlands. "For example, eating one apple a day is an easy way to increase white fruits and vegetable intake."

Reviews of randomized controlled trials have yet to show a direct link between apples and pears and heart disease risk, except for reducing body mass index — a risk factor for ticker troubles. But the most recent observational studies show apples and pears significantly lower the risk of cerebrovascular, or stroke-related, disease. How 'bout them apples?

Sweet to arteries, bitter toward plaque: How dark chocolate stacks up to stroke

Laughter may be the best medicine, but sometimes you need a dose of chocolate — so goes a popular saying. Historians think that decadent bite of ground cocoa beans has tempted people as far back as 4,000 years, and it continues to impress with health benefits today. Indulge in one of these treats every day and you could reduce your risk of stroke and open up your artery walls.

Chocolate contains flavanols like epicatechin, catechin, and procyanidins that favor your heart. Science says they may interrupt inflammation, lower blood pressure, and fend off clots that close off your arteries.

In a recent meta-analysis of 14 studies involving 508,705 people, researchers concluded that eating one to six servings of chocolate a week may be ideal for reducing the risk of stroke.

In another review, stroke risk dropped 21% for those who ate the most chocolate compared to those who ate the least. But that's no excuse to scarf down the candy aisle, say researchers. Eating more than 100 grams a week — the amount found in two chocolate snack bars — delivers enough calories, sugar, and fat to cancel out the benefits.

Make a smart choice for a smaller serving of about an ounce of dark chocolate. That's about the size of a pack of dental floss. Look for the kind with at least 70% to 85% cocoa to get the most flavanols.

Delicious ways to eat cocoa (that aren't chocolate)

The conquistadors who searched Montezuma's palace following his defeat expected to find precious metals or jewels. Instead, they found cocoa beans. For the Aztecs, cocoa was worth more than gold.

These days when people hear "cocoa," they often think "chocolate." But you can enjoy cocoa powder in a number of tasty ways. Just be sure you buy the unprocessed, natural kind because it contains the most health-promoting flavanols. Dutched cocoa, on the other hand, has been stripped of much of its nutritional benefit during processing.

- Mix a little into your yogurt, coffee, cereal, peanut butter, oatmeal, or smoothies.

- Use it in your next mole sauce to season meat.

- Whip up a batch of mocha pancakes or granola bars.

For something a little different, consider sprinkling cocoa nibs — small bits of crushed cocoa beans full of yummy chocolate flavor — into your homemade trail mix or your favorite salad.

Take a note on stroke prevention from Elvis' playbook

Apparently Elvis Presley could eat 12 to 15 grilled peanut butter banana sandwiches in one sitting. Either he truly loved the flavor or he had a serious magnesium deficiency he was trying to correct.

A single respectable version of this sandwich — one not grilled in bacon fat like Elvis preferred — on whole-wheat bread with a small banana and 2 tablespoons of unsalted chunky peanut butter satisfies 40% of the recommended daily amount of magnesium for women and 30% for men. And that's an excellent reason to add this treat to your menu.

This magnificent mineral keeps you energized and your heart rhythm normal. Plus studies show that eating more magnesium may help prevent strokes.

In one meta-analysis, people with the highest levels of magnesium were 22% less likely to have a stroke compared to those with the lowest magnesium levels.

Many reviews also agree that each additional 100 milligrams (mg) of magnesium you eat each day is linked to a 2% to 13% lower risk of stroke. That's less than the amount you'll find in the peanut butter banana sandwich or a cup of cooked spinach or black beans. Eat them throughout the day to get all 320 mg recommended for women or most of the 420 mg suggested for men.

Urinary tract infections

3 healthy ways to drown bad bacteria

Chills, fever, nausea. Most don't associate these serious symptoms with urinary tract infections (UTIs), but once you've moved past the burning, frequent urination, and pelvic pain, you are at risk for life-threatening consequences. Left untreated, the infection can spread to your kidneys and cause permanent damage. So never underestimate a UTI.

Around 40% to 60% of women have a UTI in their lifetime. And 1 in 4 suffers a repeat infection, made more likely if you've gone through menopause. That's because you have less good bacteria to combat the bad, and a hard time fully emptying your bladder. While men aren't exempt, they are at lower risk. The key to protecting yourself may be in what you drink.

With water you don't need to wish you're well. Do you limit how much you drink just to avoid frequent bathroom trips? Well, stop. You can get an infection if bad bacteria enter your urinary tract through the urethra and multiply. And a great way to keep this bacteria at bay is — you guessed it — to flush it out by drinking water.

A study in *JAMA Internal Medicine* followed 140 premenopausal women with frequent cystitis — a bladder inflammation often caused by a UTI. Researchers found that women prone to cystitis episodes halved the number of recurrences when they drank an extra 6 cups of water each day for a year.

Green tea shuts down bad bacteria. "Thank God for tea!" wrote Sydney Smith, preacher and founder of the prestigious British periodical *The Edinburgh Review*.

Eat	
Kefir	Cranberry juice
Water	Green tea

Avoid
Caffeine
Alcohol
Acidic drinks

"What would the world do without tea! How did it exist?" Fortunately, you don't have to imagine a world without tea — which is good news if you suffer from UTIs.

Natural compounds in green tea are known to fight bad bacteria. So researchers at Oakland University William Beaumont School of Medicine examined the effects of green tea extract on UTI-causing bacteria — specifically *E.coli*. They found the polyphenols in green tea, especially epicatechin-3-gallate (ECG), kept the bacteria from growing.

Drinking just 1 cup of green tea could positively affect the bacteria in your urinary tract, and several cups throughout the day could provide long-lasting protection.

All you've heard about cranberries is true. Not all old wives' tales hold up against science, but cranberries for UTIs is one exception. Canadian researchers discovered a cranberry extract had some big benefits.

- It allowed antibiotics to enter bacteria cells more easily.

- It disrupted the process bacteria use to get rid of antibiotics.

- It prevented the bacteria from developing a resistance to the antibiotics.

That means doctors can use a lower dose of antibiotics to treat UTIs.

While cranberries may help prevent UTIs and boost the power of your medication, they can't treat an active UTI by themselves. Still, many experts urge you to try cranberry products, like powder capsules and sugar-free juices, especially if you have a history of recurring, uncomplicated UTIs.

> UTIs may affect parts of the urinary system beyond your bladder. But more shocking is they can increase your risk of ischemic stroke — the kind where an artery to the brain is blocked. Strokes can be triggered by all sorts of infections, and in the case of UTIs, a new study found they triple the risk of an ischemic stroke in the 30 days following infection.

Find it fresh: Handy hints help you buy and store cranberries

Want to add cranberries to your diet? Follow these smart shopping and storing tips for best results.

Fresh cranberries float and bounce, but since you can't do that at the store, you'll have to rely on sight and touch.

- Check the color. The shade of red won't matter when it comes to taste, but a deeper color means they are packed with more nutrients. Avoid ones that have brown spots.

- Check the texture. Skip shriveled berries and feel through the bag for mushiness. Make sure there's no liquid in the bag either.

Once you get them home, take out any shriveled or brown berries you missed. Store the rest in a tightly sealed plastic bag in your fridge for a month. If they feel sticky or tough when you take them out, they've gone bad and it's time to toss them. They'll keep for a year in your freezer.

Don't flare your symptoms — dodge these irritating drinks

Not all liquids are created equal when it comes to UTIs. Although most any fluid will flush out bacteria, avoid acidic drinks, caffeine, and alcohol. They can irritate your bladder and worsen your UTI symptoms.

- Acidic drinks like juice, especially orange and lemon, may cause bladder irritation by changing the pH of your urine. Originally, scientists thought acidic urine helped kill bad bacteria. But a recent study shows that less acidic urine actually prevents bacterial growth better. Cranberry juice is the exception here because its powers against bacteria outweigh the negative effects of its acidity.

- Caffeine is a diuretic — it causes your kidneys to make more urine and helps you get rid of extra fluid and salt. So it can intensify an urge to go to the bathroom.

- Alcohol can increase the acidity of your urine and worsen symptoms. It may have other side effects if mixed with antibiotics for UTIs.

Urinary tract problems? Drink this milk right away

Getting rid of a urinary tract infection may not be as easy as simply exchanging bad bacteria for the good kind. But some research suggests you can push past UTIs by adding more of the good kind — in the form of probiotics — to your diet. And one of the easiest and most effective ways to do that is with a probiotic drink.

Probiotics beat your bladder troubles. With so many health drinks crowding the market, you may not have heard of kefir. But if you get UTIs, it could be your new best friend.

Kefir, pronounced kuh-FEAR, is a probiotic-rich fermented milk drink made with kefir grains, which are not really grains at all, but small masses of friendly lactic acid bacteria and acetic acid bacteria. These bacteria are known to improve your intestinal tract and immune system health. Plus they reduce recurring incidences of UTI. How? Two ways.

- Probiotics prevent bad bacteria from attaching to urinary tract cells.

- They change your urine's pH to make it harder for bacteria to grow.

A dairy-free dose of probiotics gets rid of UTIs. When it ferments, kefir turns much, but not all, of milk's natural sugars, called lactose, into lactic acid. However, if you want a totally lactose-free drink, you can buy water kefir. This is completely dairy-free and is made with sugar water, fruit juice, or coconut water.

Instead of tasting like tangy yogurt, water kefir has a sweet, slightly fermented flavor and can be jazzed up with fruit, extracts, or herbs. Since you're wanting the probiotics, not necessarily the calcium, you'll still get the lactic acid-producing bacteria you need to fight a UTI.

Looking for other nondairy probiotic options? Try sauerkraut, kombucha, and miso.

Remember, probiotics aren't an alternative to antibiotics prescribed by your doctor, but they may be helpful.

The wonder herb that fights off infection

Good news for garlic lovers everywhere — this flavor-enhancing food may help your bladder, too.

Allicin is a compound produced when you chop or crush garlic. It doesn't just give garlic its characteristically pungent smell. Along with other sulfur compounds, it's the force behind garlic's antimicrobial punch. In fact, garlic's effect even holds up against bacteria that has become drug-resistant.

In a study out of India's Birla Institute of Technology and Sciences, garlic extract faced off against 166 bacteria strains isolated from the urine of people with urinary tract infections. Scientists found that over 80% of the antibiotic-resistant bacteria they tested was impacted by the garlic.

Although this is still early research, garlic may turn out to be one spicy way to fight UTIs.

Weight gain

Fullness factor — get a leg up with legumes

Have you packed on more pounds than you'd like to admit? You're probably taking in more calories than you're burning off. It's easy to do if you eat too many processed foods that leave you hungry shortly after eating.

Want to feel fuller for longer periods of time? Add these nutritious legumes to your plate.

Pack in protein the easy, peas-y way. Your body needs protein to build and repair tissue. But instead of tucking into a steak, why not turn to beans and peas? Danish researchers compared the fullness factor of 43 men who ate high-protein breakfasts containing either beans and peas or veal and pork. The men who ate the legumes reported feeling fuller after eating and later ate 12% fewer calories at lunch.

The researchers say the high fiber content of the beans and peas — four times that of the meat-based meals — probably satisfied the men's hunger for longer. Looking for more protein-packed, high-fiber legumes? Try navy beans, kidney beans, and chickpeas.

Load up on lentils to lose body fat. This Biblical food can be a saving grace. Just 1 cup of cooked lentils contains a whopping 18 grams of protein. That's 36% of your daily requirement.

So how does all that protein help you lose weight? Compared with fats and carbohydrates, protein triggers the greatest release in your gut of a hunger-squashing hormone called peptide YY, or PYY. The end result — you eat less and feel full after feasting on lentils. This can

Eat

Olive oil	Nuts
Kumquats	Blueberries
Ginger	Oolong tea
Rooibos tea	Oatmeal
Peas	Lentils
Peanut butter	Safflower oil

Avoid

Sugary beverages like soda and fruit drinks

Processed foods

help you drop pounds and lower your body fat, according to a study in the *American Journal of Clinical Nutrition.*

Remember to rinse your lentils of any dust or debris before boiling. Lentils don't require soaking like other legumes.

Partake of peanuts to lower blood sugar. Did you know peanuts aren't really nuts? They're actually considered legumes. Real nuts grow on trees, but peanuts are edible seeds that grow on pods underground. Another important difference? They're not as expensive as tree nuts, and a small study says they may satisfy your hunger pangs.

The research on obese women at risk for developing diabetes found that just over 2 1/2 tablespoons of creamy peanut butter in the morning can curb hunger all day. The volunteers were divided into three groups and shared a common breakfast of orange juice and Cream of Wheat breakfast porridge followed by a high-carbohydrate lunch of bread and strawberry jam.

> Can a hidden food intolerance make you fat? Some experts think so. The theory is that food sensitivities cause inflammation, which leads to weight gain. Talk to your doctor if you suspect a problem. In some studies, participants had difficulty losing weight until they began a diet plan customized from results of a food sensitivity test.

- The first group added 1 1/2 ounces of peanuts to their breakfast.

- The second added the same amount of peanut butter.

- The third, a control group, added nothing to their meals.

Compared with the control group, the women who ate the peanut butter and peanuts had higher concentrations of PYY in their systems after eating and a lower desire to eat for up to 12 hours after breakfast.

Just keep an eye on your peanut butter portion. Because it's a calorie-dense, high-fat food, many experts recommend you stick to a standard serving size of 2 tablespoons.

The whole truth: Eat these grains for a slimmer silhouette

A diet rich in whole grains — the kind that contain 100% of the original kernel — has been shown to ward off major illnesses like heart disease, high blood pressure, and colon cancer. They even help stabilize your blood sugar, lower your cholesterol, protect your eyesight in old age, and reduce your risk of gallstones.

One reason why? They're natural "good carbs" loaded with protein, fiber, B vitamins, antioxidants, and trace minerals. Unlike refined grains — think white rice and white flour — whole grains haven't been stripped of their nutritious bran and germ. And that may prove key when it comes to weight loss.

Boost metabolism with whole grains. Past studies suggest whole grains help reduce belly and total body fat. Recent research sheds light on how.

Scientists at Tufts University divided 81 adults into two groups and fed them a similar diet for two weeks. Then, the participants were randomly assigned to eat either whole grains or refined grains over the next six weeks. Otherwise, their diets were similar. Here's what the scientists found at the end of the study.

> At least half the grains you eat should be whole grains, according to the U.S. Department of Agriculture. You can increase the amount you get by adding whole-wheat pasta and bread, brown rice, barley, and whole-grain cereal to your menu. Other tasty whole grains include quinoa, buckwheat, and popcorn.

- Those who ate the whole grains experienced an increase in their resting metabolic rate. That's the total number of calories your body burns at rest.

- The whole-grain eaters lost more calories in their stool. That's because the calories in the fiber of whole grains aren't fully absorbed.

The combination of those two factors added up to nearly 100 calories a day. The researchers say that translates into a loss of 5 1/2 pounds over the course of a year.

Stop weight gain with oatmeal. If you eat just one thing for breakfast, make it this superfood. After all, nutrient-packed oatmeal reduces hunger. That's according to the findings of a small study comparing the fullness factor of adults who ate a breakfast of either cereal or oatmeal. Both meals had the same amount of calories.

The researchers found that the participants felt less hungry over the four hours after eating an oatmeal breakfast, which is higher in fiber and protein but lower in sugar than cereal. The scientists think oatmeal's appetite-controlling properties come from beta glucan, a form of soluble fiber that may also improve digestion because it increases the amount of time food stays in your intestines. That's important because slower digestion leaves you feeling fuller longer and less likely to snack.

You'll be bowled over by this new take on instant oatmeal

Delicious and nutritious oats come in many varieties like steel cut, rolled, and old-fashioned. But on a busy morning they take too long to cook. Instant oat packets are speedy, but they're full of sugar and artificial sweeteners. And they're triple the price. Save time and money with this "oat-standing" recipe.

In your blender, combine 1 cup old-fashioned oats, 1 tablespoon brown sugar (optional), 1/2 teaspoon cinnamon, and 1/2 teaspoon salt. Blend on medium until oats are powdered. Add 2 more cups of oats and "pulse" your blender until the oats are broken down. Store the mixture in an airtight container for up to three months. Makes six servings.

Ready to enjoy your oatmeal? Just pour 1/2 cup mixture in a bowl with 3/4 cup of boiling water. Stir, then let stand for one minute. Add your favorite toppings — think dried fruit and chopped nuts — and enjoy.

Sip yourself slim with 2 tasty teas

It's said in China that drinking a daily cup of tea will surely starve the pharmacist. It's no wonder, considering tea contains compounds linked to a lower risk of developing serious medical conditions like cancer, diabetes, and heart disease.

Research also suggests a mug of soothing tea can get you closer to your weight loss goals.

Oolong tea zaps fat cells. Chinese scientists wanted to look at the effects of oolong tea on body weight. So they recruited 102 overweight or obese adults and had them drink almost 1 1/2 cups of oolong tea four times a day.

- After six weeks, over half of them lost more than 2 pounds without significantly changing their diets.

- Some of the severely obese participants lost even more — over 6 1/2 pounds.

- As an added bonus, some of the participants also experienced drops in their cholesterol and triglyceride numbers.

The researchers say catechins — flavonoid compounds with antioxidant properties — may have prevented the growth of new fat cells and absorption of fats from the intestine.

Rooibos tea boosts your metabolism. Research suggests that drinking rooibos tea may help you lose weight. South African scientists experimenting with cell cultures found that polyphenol compounds in rooibos tea lowered the formation of fat cells by a whopping 22%. They also found that the micronutrients increased the rate at which fats are broken down and used for energy.

A spoonful of sugar may help the medicine go down, but it can also make the scale go up. Want a quick fix? Animal research shows honey causes less weight gain than common sugar. Try it in your tea instead of sugar to sweeten the deal of these already helpful hot drinks.

Never heard of rooibos tea? It's a red, caffeine-free tea made from the leaves of a shrub grown on the western coast of South Africa. The sweet-tasting tea has grown in popularity in the U.S., so you can easily find it in grocery stores.

Weight loss stalled?
Root out the problem with ginger

Want to boost your metabolism and block your body's absorption of fat? Then head over to your spice rack for some ginger.

That would be the advice of Iranian researchers who divided obese women into two groups. Half ate 2 grams of ginger powder — about a heaping teaspoon — daily over 12 weeks. The rest took a placebo. Three months later, the ginger group saw a significant reduction in their body mass index (BMI) compared with the control group.

Why is your BMI important? It's a good indication of how much fat you're carrying around. People with a high BMI run a greater risk of developing high blood pressure, heart disease, and other conditions.

The scientists say ginger helps you burn more calories. In addition, it may help you meet your weight goals by blocking an enzyme your gut uses to absorb fats from food.

3 smart tips to whittle your middle

A poor diet. Physical inactivity. A slowing metabolism. Add 'em up and you're looking at a recipe for middle-age spread. Call it what you will — Buddha belly, muffin top, or spare tire — there's no escaping the fact that extra weight tends to collect in the midsection after a certain age.

Been packing on some extra pounds? These foods will help slam the brakes on a problematic paunch.

Banish bulge with nonsugary drinks. That's according to researchers who examined the drinking habits of some 1,000 participants in the Framingham Heart Study. The middle-aged volunteers had their abdominal fat measured once at the beginning of the study and again six years later.

The results? The participants who had at least one sugar-sweetened drink a day gained 27% more deep belly fat — the kind that's linked to diabetes and heart disease — than those who rarely, if ever, drank sugary refreshments like soda and fruit drinks. The researchers say the excess sugar may trigger insulin resistance and increase the amount of fat stored in your abdomen.

Cook with safflower oil to find a flatter tummy. Research published in *Clinical Nutrition* and the *American Journal of Clinical Nutrition* indicates this amazing oil helps belly fat slide right off your middle, even if you have a lot to lose.

The study of obese women with diabetes found that adding just 1 2/3 teaspoons a day of safflower oil to their diets helped them lose up to 4 pounds of abdominal fat in four months. The women, all of them seniors who didn't alter their diets in any other way, even added an average of up to 3 pounds of muscle and improved their cholesterol and blood sugar levels.

Safflower oil is rich in healthy fats called polyunsaturated fatty acids, which the researchers believe contributed to the results of the study.

Combat midlife midriff with blueberries. Surprising research suggests this tiny fruit contains compounds that reduce belly fat.

Scientists at the University of Michigan divided obesity-prone rats into groups and fed them either high-fat or low-fat foods. Both diets were mixed with either blueberry powder or a placebo. Amazingly, after three months the rats on the high-fat meal plan with blueberry powder lost belly fat and experienced health benefits like lower triglycerides and improved insulin sensitivity.

But that doesn't mean you should go hog wild on fatty foods. The rats on the low-fat diet with blueberry powder saw the same results, but with the additional benefits of significantly reduced body weight, liver weight, and total body fat.

Researchers say anthocyanins — the antioxidant-rich pigments in blueberries that give them their color — may change how your body stores and processes sugar.

'A nutter' way to rein in weight gain

Nutty about nuts? Then you'll enjoy this little quiz. Which nut is a cousin to poison ivy? Cashews. An itchy oil hides in their shell. What ancient civilization believed hazelnuts could cure baldness? Greece, naturally. No bald deities on Mount Olympus. Now here's a tough one — what nuts are going to help you lose weight? All of them!

Shell-shocking news about nuts. Studies have found that eating a small portion of nuts regularly may protect you from packing on extra pounds.

In fact, experts say replacing just half a serving per day of unhealthy foods — like cookies, chips, cake, or red and processed meat — with a handful of your favorite nuts may be just the ticket for preventing middle-age spread. Researchers found that eating as little as 1/2 ounce every day is linked to less weight gain and a lower risk of obesity. How's that for nut appeal?

How it works — in a nutshell. Experts say the reason nuts are so great for your weight may be threefold.

- Chomping a handful of nuts takes some effort, which may lead you to eat less.

- The high fiber content of nuts delays stomach emptying, so you feel satisfied longer. Plus the fiber binds to fats in your gut, so more calories are removed through the processes of digestion.

- Evidence shows that the unsaturated fat in nuts may cause you to burn more calories while you're at rest.

What nut should you crack to get the best results? How about a dozen almonds or maybe 10 walnuts? Actually, any nut will do. Just don't go overboard. Remember, even small portions of nuts are high in fat and calories. Check the label before you dig in. And for the healthiest option, choose plain, unsalted nuts.

Kumquats: A bite-sized fruit with fat-fighting powers

Want to lose weight? Then try eating kumquats — the oval-shaped fruit with an oddball name. This low-cal treat is packed with lots of belly-filling fiber and has little to no fat, sodium, or cholesterol. What's more, scientists have discovered these fruits contain a nutrient that shows tremendous promise in battling the bulge.

Those are the findings of Canadian researchers who fed mice either a high-fat diet or a high-fat diet that contained naringenin, a flavonoid found in citrus fruits like kumquats. After four weeks, the scientists found that the naringenin-fed group didn't gain nearly as much weight as the control mice. They say the addition of naringenin caused the mice's livers to burn fat instead of store it.

Not so sure if you've ever eaten a kumquat? It's golden orange in color and about the size of a cherry tomato. The sweetness of its skin, rich in essential oils, offsets the sourness of a juicy pulp. You'll want to eat the peel — that's where most of the naringenin is found.

Here's another reason to dig into kumquats and other citrus fruits. They're chock-full of other flavonoids that are kind to your waistline. A study on the diets of 2,734 healthy female twins found that the women who ate the most flavonoids had significantly less body fat than those who got the least. Other good sources of citrus flavonoids include grapefruits, limes, lemons, and oranges.

Order up veggies to stem weight gain

Imagine you had the chance to invite singer Paul McCartney and boxer Mike Tyson over for dinner. What a night that would be. But what would you serve them?

Seems like such different men would have very different tastes indeed. But if truth be told, your guests would probably pick tofu and quinoa over a grilled T-bone. Why? Because they understand the benefits of a vegetarian diet.

So how could retreating from meat help you? A study recently published in the journal *Nutrients* gives some insight.

Sidestep the spare tire by going vegetarian. The 10-year Spanish study of 16,000 university graduates found that those who ate a vegetarian diet were less likely to become obese as years passed compared to folks who favored meatier meals.

At the start of the study, participants filled out detailed food questionnaires that awarded them points according to the amount of plant foods — fruits, vegetables, grains, legumes, olive oil, and nuts — they ate each day. Points were taken off for animal fats, dairy, eggs, fish, seafood, and meat. The participants were then divided into five groups based on their total scores.

At the end of the study, the researchers discovered that people with the most pro-vegetarian diets were 43% less likely to become obese compared to those who ate the most animal foods.

Why do plant-eaters tend to be slimmer? Experts believe they've gotten to the root of the matter. For one, all the fiber and phyto-chemicals found in fruits and veggies are kind to your waistline, while the high-calorie saturated fat found in meat is not.

In addition, some doctors think vegetarians may pay more attention to other areas of their health, not just their diet. For instance, they may exercise more and smoke less.

The authors of the Spanish study boiled their findings down to this. "Plant-based diets are associated with substantially lower risk of developing obesity. This supports current recommendations to shift to diets rich in plant foods, with lower intake of animal foods."

Couple healthier living with healthier eating, and you're one step closer to hanging on to that slim, trim figure for life.

Unexplained weight loss?
How to tip the scales in your favor

Are you shedding pounds without even trying? Don't do a happy dance just yet. Unexplained weight loss — losing 5% of your normal body weight in six months to a year without trying — could point to a health problem and jeopardize your independence. So see your doctor if you're losing inches and don't know why. Meanwhile, you can boost your calorie count with these healthy tips.

- Try eating five or six small meals instead of three large meals.

- Eat starchy vegetables like corn and potatoes and dense fruits like bananas and raisins.

- Add shredded cheese to salads, soups, and casseroles.

- Drizzle olive oil over vegetables to boost flavor and calories.

- Prepare cream soups and hot cereals with whole milk instead of water.

Eat like a Greek to keep the pounds off

Can 2,000 years of history be wrong? Not according to the trim folks following the traditional eating style of Italians, Greeks, and others living along the Mediterranean Sea. Fortunately, you don't have to travel farther than your supermarket to eat like you're living in one of these coastal countries.

Melt away extra pounds by digging into delish dishes. Diverse flavors surround the Mediterranean, but the menus are rooted in the same healthy foundation. People on the Mediterranean diet avoid unhealthy fats and sweets and favor fish, fruits, and vegetables over meat. Foods like olive oil, nuts, yogurt, and whole grains are staples, too.

And if this diet's centuries-long list of supporters doesn't sway you, researchers recently set out to determine just how much of an impact changing to a Mediterranean diet can have. In an eight-week study, the scientists found that the Mediterranean diet can improve weight loss and cholesterol levels. That means it drops the risk of heart disease, too.

But if you think you can make a few swaps and reap all the rewards, think again. Just adding a few Mediterranean foods to your normal fare isn't enough. At the end of the two months, people who switched to an entirely Mediterranean diet lost more weight than those who either added some typical Mediterranean foods to their meals or stayed with their Western diet.

Avoid overeating to keep your scale happy. Healthy food isn't all the Mediterranean diet offers. It also helps curb the urge to overindulge, say researchers of a small animal study. They fed animals either a Western or Mediterranean diet and allowed them to eat as much as they wanted.

"What we found was that the group on the Mediterranean diet actually ate fewer calories, had lower body weight, and had less body fat than those on the Western diet," said the study's principal investigator, Carol A. Shively, Ph.D., professor of pathology at Wake Forest School of Medicine.

A Western diet is designed to be "hyperpalatable" — the foods make you want to eat more. That's partly because the refined carbs in processed food spike then plummet your blood sugar, leaving you yearning for another snack instead of feeling full.

The Mediterranean diet, on the other hand, is packed with fiber and healthy fats that fill you up without encouraging you to overeat. Eureka!

Olive oil: A wonder food for staving off hunger

A Mediterranean diet wouldn't be complete without a healthy dose of its "secret sauce" — olive oil. Great in dressings, stir-fries, and marinades, it's also good for your heart and belly.

You probably already know olive oil contains monounsaturated fatty acids (MUFAs), a fat that helps keep your arteries clear of cholesterol plaques. But did you know a particular MUFA called oleic acid also turns off hunger pangs between meals?

According to a University of California study on rats, oleic acid sparks the production of a hunger-fighting compound — dubbed oleoylethanolamide — that indirectly signals feelings of fullness to your brain.

Just be sure to exercise portion control. Although olive oil is low in cholesterol and sodium, it's calorie dense. A single tablespoon, for example, has 119 calories.

Is it time to keep or kick the keto diet?

What do basketball legend LeBron James, journalist Katie Couric, and Oscar-winning actress Halle Berry have in common? They've all sung praises for the low-carbohydrate, high-fat ketogenic diet. Could this food trend be right for you?

The carb crackdown zeroes in on fat. This diet means drastically cutting the amount of carbs you eat — think bread, pasta, cereal, and juice — and replacing them with healthy fats from foods like avocado, grass-fed meat, olive oil, nuts, and seeds.

Typically, 55% of the American diet is devoted to carbs, but that plummets to 10% or less on the keto diet. The lack of carbs puts your body into ketosis, a metabolic state where you burn fat for fuel instead of glucose. This lets the weight slip off — as much as 10 pounds in just two weeks, though some of that will be water weight.

Doctors first started using this diet almost 100 years ago to treat epilepsy. And now, along with weight loss, new research suggests it could help with type 2 diabetes. That's because minimizing carbs keeps blood sugar levels at a low but healthy level.

Balance your diet for best health benefits. Fans of the keto diet enjoy eating as much low-carb food as they want. After all, who wants to count calories? But the limited food choice means you'll likely miss out on important nutrients. And in the first few weeks you may face side effects like fatigue and dizziness that can make the diet difficult to stick to.

Oddly enough, keeping the diet brief may be a good thing. Scientists aren't certain of the diet's long-term effects. But they have come up with a possible compromise.

Researchers have found that two short periods on the keto eating plan — separated by longer periods of sticking to the more balanced Mediterranean diet — leads to successful long-term weight loss and other health benefits. In the study, the keto phases were 20 days and the Mediterranean phases lasted at least four months, but talk with your doctor before making any major diet changes.

Index